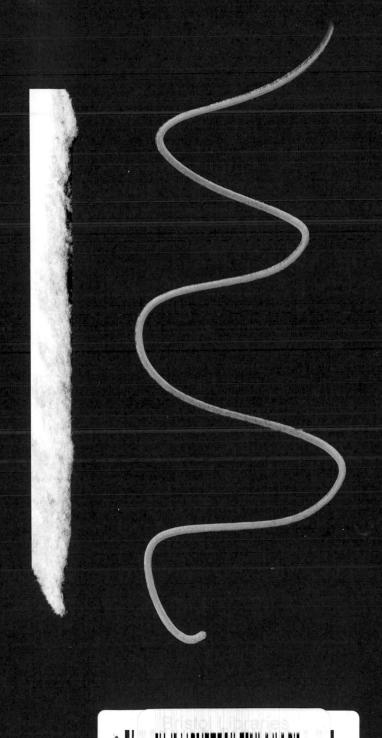

FAT, FATE, AND DISEASE

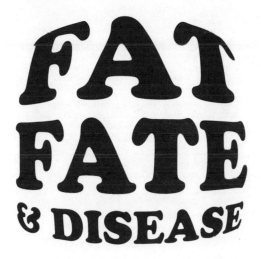

FAT FATE & DISEASE

Why exercise and diet are not enough

PETER GLUCKMAN
& MARK HANSON

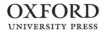

OXFORD
UNIVERSITY PRESS

OXFORD

UNIVERSITY PRESS

Great Clarendon Street, Oxford OX2 6DP

Oxford University Press is a department of the University of Oxford.
It furthers the University's objective of excellence in research, scholarship,
and education by publishing worldwide in

Oxford New York

Auckland Cape Town Dar es Salaam Hong Kong Karachi
Kuala Lumpur Madrid Melbourne Mexico City Nairobi
New Delhi Shanghai Taipei Toronto

With offices in

Argentina Austria Brazil Chile Czech Republic France Greece
Guatemala Hungary Italy Japan Poland Portugal Singapore
South Korea Switzerland Thailand Turkey Ukraine Vietnam

Oxford is a registered trade mark of Oxford University Press
in the UK and in certain other countries

Published in the United States
by Oxford University Press Inc., New York

British Library Cataloguing in Publication Data

Data available

Library of Congress Cataloging in Publication Data

Library of Congress Control Number: 2011942638

Typeset by SPI Publisher Services, Pondicherry, India
Printed in Great Britain
on acid-free paper by
Clays Ltd, St Ives plc

ISBN 978–0–19–964462–9

1 3 5 7 9 10 8 6 4 2

Contents

Acknowledgements

Our professional lives have been occupied with the study of development in early life, both before and after birth, and of how different patterns of development affect our health in both the short and the long term. Our research has focused not just on the mechanisms underlying these relationships, but also on the larger question of *why* our early development is so plastic. The implications of this research for understanding the human condition are substantial. As our research progressed, we thought increasingly about the mismatch between the way evolution has moulded our biology and the world we have created. Our fundamental biology appears to be at odds with our contemporary world. Although both are parts of our 'normal' lives, they have consequences which are reflected in the growing burden of the so-called non-communicable diseases—especially diabetes, cardiovascular disease, and the associated condition of obesity.

As we talked these ideas over, we realized that they were not widely appreciated, and were not incorporated into current strategies to reduce the burden of non-communicable diseases. In fact the reverse seemed to be true—the relevance of early developmental life to the risk of later disease seemed to be side-lined, just as developmental biology had been in biological and medical science for much of the 20th century. In addition, despite the fact that current strategies to reduce non-communicable disease met with limited success in many situations, there appeared to be a stubborn adherence to an inappropriate medical model of these diseases, as if we were viewing them in the same way as infectious diseases. The strategy seemed to be directed at treating those adults who already have the disease—at least in societies where such treatment can be afforded—and trying to isolate individuals from the causative agents, namely smoking, dietary sugar, salt and fat, and sedentary behaviour.

For despite all the efforts of public health and of medical science to promote healthy lifestyles, the problems of diabetes, heart disease, and obesity continue to grow. Similar trends exist for some allergic and immune disorders and lung disease. The Western world gets fatter and the diet industry richer. And now the problem is exploding in the developing world too—there are hundreds of millions of people who now have diabetes or heart disease, even though many of them are not obese by Western standards. Many of them are young adults, although traditionally these are diseases of middle age. But it is also apparent, as we look at developing countries, that the solution requires attention from not just a medical perspective but a much broader developmental agenda. The more we thought about this, the more we realized that clearly something is missing from our strategy, because we are not winning the war against these diseases.

We started to communicate our concerns about this omission in lectures at conferences and in academic articles. Some of our scientific colleagues welcomed the intercession, others seemed uninterested or even resistant. The more we pursued the implications of the ideas, the more we felt the presence of vested interests in various forms, which operated to limit their inclusion in current strategy formation. What seemed increasingly obvious to us was sometimes met with denial as well as incomprehension. We began to feel like the little boy who cried 'The emperor has no clothes!' His statement of what everyone knew but did not want to admit produced a social change, although not so much through a direct effect on the emperor's deceitful courtiers as from the public reaction which followed his outburst. This book is our cry.

Given the many years and the multiple dimensions of our research, there are many people who have wittingly or unwittingly influenced our thinking. Many of them encouraged us in pursuing what was clearly an unpopular set of ideas. First we must acknowledge the colleagues, research fellows, and students with whom we have worked most recently, including Alan Beedle, Tatjana Buklijas, Felicia Low, Mark Vickers, Deb Sloboda, Tony Pleasants, Wayne Cutfield, Allan Sheppard (Auckland); Chong Yap Seng, Michael Meaney, Ravi Khambadur, Melvin Leow, Lee Yung Seng, Emilia Tng, Tai E. Shyong (Singapore); Keith Godfrey, Cyrus Cooper, Karen Lillycrop, Graham Burdge, Philip Calder, Christopher Byrne, Lucy Green, Kirsten Poore, Felino Cagampang, Rohan Lewis, Christopher Torrens, Geraldine Clough, Hazel Inskip, Caroline Fall, Nick Harvey, Aven Ahie-Sayer, Richard Oreffo, Kim Bruce, Jane Cleal, Sîan Robinson, Elaine Dennison (Southampton). Felicia and Tatjana also helped with some research for the manuscript.

We are very grateful to Terrence Forrester in Jamaica, Ronald Ma in Hong Kong, Alex Ferraro in Sao Paolo, Huixia Yang in Beijing, Tony Duan in Shanghai, Torvid Kiserud in Bergen and Ethiopia, Guttorm Haugen in Oslo, John Newnham in Perth, Australia, Anibal Llanos in Santiago de Chile, and Carlos Blanco in Dublin for their collegiality and scientific insights and for giving us important perspectives into problems in parts of the world they know well.

We have had informal discussions with many colleagues including Steve Simpson (Sydney), David Raubenheimer (Auckland), Paul Zimmet (Melbourne), John Funder (Melbourne), Pat Bateson (Cambridge), Randy Nesse (Ann Arbor), Carl Bergstrom (Seattle), Craig Rubens (Seattle), Hamish Spencer and Peter Dearden (Otago), James Heckman and Chris Kuzawa (Chicago), Tessa Roseboom (Amsterdam), and several scientists active in the nutrition and pharmaceutical industries.

We are indebted to Jane Kitcher (Southampton) and Megan Jeffries (Auckland), who cheerfully produced corrected versions of the book throughout its gestation, often at short notice. This is the fourth book we have written together, and yet again we thank our families for their forbearance in putting up with our distracted behaviour and frequent absences.

Peter Gluckman and Mark Hanson
Auckland, Southampton, and places in between
May 2011

1

Blinkers and Biases

What seems to be the problem?

Only 2,000 years ago our planet housed fewer than 300 million people, 100 years ago it was home to 1.5 billion, and now there are about seven billion of us. And we will potentially add at least another two billion to the world population over the next 40 years. Most of that growth will occur in the developing and least developed world, where much of the population is young, compared with the ageing populations of the developed world. For the first time in our history more than half of us live in cities rather than in rural areas and this shift to urban living is set to go on increasing. There is massive economic productivity and continuing growth in the world, even though it has stumbled a little in the past few years, but many of us are still incredibly poor— living on less than US$1 a day—and this number will increase too. From the lowest-income societies to the vast developing economies such as India and China, we are seeing enormous social changes. Along with economic development a big change is taking place in what people eat and how they live their lives.

All these global inhabitants will have to be fed and need access to safer food and clean water, hygienic living conditions, and a supply of energy. Energy supplies drive economic growth and we have become increasingly concerned about where that energy is going to come from in the near future. Our reliance on fossil fuels such as coal and oil leads to greenhouse gas emissions, as do the destruction of forests and the expansion of agriculture needed to sustain our expanding population. And so the world heats up.

This crisis of depletion of non-renewable energy supplies, of climate change, of degrading and uncertain water supplies, and of growing insecurity in the world's food supply has been called 'the perfect storm' by the UK government's chief scientist Sir John Beddington. This storm is a direct result of the ever-increasing number of humans living on a planet which does not have infinite resources: a population increase which in turn reflects the many ways in which we humans have changed our world.

Many of us are becoming increasingly concerned about how we can survive this storm, at least with a way of life which meets our aspirations and expectations. This issue of the quality of life for all of us forms the backdrop for this book, but our concerns extend much further than that. We have changed the planet, but we have also changed ourselves—not in the fundamental biological processes that make our bodies work, because they took millions of years to evolve and so cannot change quickly, but we have dramatically changed what we eat, the way we work, the way we expend energy, and the very pattern of our lives. More and more of us use cars instead of walking to get around; we work at a keyboard rather than at hard manual labour; and we live much longer lives than our ancestors. Many of us have smaller families and, at least in the West, many women have their first baby at a much older age than their grandmothers or even their mothers.

The consequences of these changes in the way we live leave us with a fundamental discrepancy with our biology—a *mismatch*. And this mismatch has consequences which will make Sir John's 'storm' look even more frightening and urgent. The storm clouds are darker and deeper than we had realized, because they herald another tempest, one that threatens our health and much more. For many of us around the world striving to have better lives, it will undermine our chance of doing so.

Most of us, if asked about today's major global health problems, would focus on HIV-AIDS, on the risk of a flu pandemic, on malaria, and maybe even on polio or tuberculosis. Some of us might refer to dengue fever and other tropical diseases, which are common in many developing countries but unfamiliar to many of us in the West. These infectious, or communicable, diseases cause an enormous burden of death and suffering across the world and have been the major focus of campaigns funded by organizations such as the Bill and Melinda Gates Foundation. But this book goes beyond the challenges of infectious disease. We are writing about health issues that are even more pressing. There is urgency to what we will discuss, partly because it has not been sufficiently recognized but also because new health problems, which are emerging quickly, may take more than a generation to fix and so we cannot afford to delay doing something about them.

The health issues which this book is about are the so-called non-communicable diseases—the major ones being cardiovascular disease (heart attacks, strokes, high blood pressure), diabetes, cancer, and lung disease. Other non-communicable diseases are linked to these—kidney and bowel disease, bone and joint disease, skin disease, asthma, some forms of blindness, mental and cognitive disorders . . . the list soon becomes extensive. Together these diseases account for more than 36 million deaths every year—that is nearly two-thirds of all global deaths. These deaths are premature, in other words they kill many of us when we are still in our prime, possibly even when we are young, and they are certainly not just problems of old age.

On an optimistic note, these diseases are preventable, which means we don't have to accept this dreadful death toll. However, nearly 80 per cent of these diseases occur in low- and middle-income countries—developing countries where the resources to prevent them scarcely exist.

In this book we will focus largely on two of these non-communicable diseases which are of growing concern everywhere, namely, diabetes and cardiovascular disease. These diseases are closely linked, and in general when we talk about non-communicable diseases in this book this is what we mean. One of the reasons why the problem which these non-communicable diseases pose is not sufficiently recognized is that we might not automatically link them together. If they occurred individually they might be tackled one by one. But they don't—and herein lies much of the problem. Many of the reasons as to why we develop diabetes and cardiovascular disease also underlie some forms of cancer and other non-communicable diseases.

A related problem is that these diseases generally do not kill us straight away—they emerge slowly and subtly and do not create the emotional impact of malaria or HIV-AIDS (someone is either HIV-positive or they are not). Indeed, because diabetes and cardiovascular disease are perceived as being a result of how we each live our lives—almost part of normal life, some might say—the collective ownership by society of the problems they create is often not recognized or is played down. We will explain why we cannot continue to think in this way.

When we write about diabetes in this book we are not referring to the well-known type 1 diabetes of young people, which is thought to be due to the destruction of the insulin-making cells of the pancreas by the body's own immune system, but rather to type 2 diabetes, which used to be called 'maturity onset diabetes'. This has a different biological basis and is largely due to insulin not working sufficiently well in the liver and muscle for a person to control their blood sugar levels. It is linked to obesity because this makes it harder for insulin to work, and to cardio-vascular disease because the metabolic disturbances of the disease inter-fere with blood vessel and heart function.

We will not focus on the diseases themselves in the book—this is not a medical book. Nor will we burden the reader with unnecessary jargon or technical information. Our purpose is to go beyond them to understand *why* they occur, *why* they are becoming much more common, and *why* we are failing so badly in our attempts to deal with them. We will argue that collectively we have misunderstood the nature of the problem. We have been fighting the wrong enemies in our war on these diseases and this has led us to use the wrong strategies. If we are to win this war we need to undertake some urgent rethinking about the real foes we face and what our strategy should be.

In addition to the personal and family tragedies which non-communicable diseases cause, economists calculate that if unchecked they will cost the global economy far more than the infectious diseases, more than many conflicts. The World Economic Forum calculates that in global risk terms they rank with climate change or a global financial meltdown as a major threat to human society and the way we live.

The doctor's dilemma

Doctors, health ministries, and philanthropic organizations are becoming increasingly aware of the challenge of non-communicable diseases and are trying to deal with it. But they are coming to it rather late in the day. It is only now that they recognize what an enormous problem it represents in the developing world as well as in the devel-oped world. We will contend that they largely have a mistaken idea of what needs to be done. Their current range of interventions are poorly focused, incomplete, and inadequate.

A medical problem is far easier to tackle if we know what causes it. When we first understood in 1982 that AIDS was a communicable disease, the hunt began for the agent which was responsible for it. Once the HIV virus had been identified it was easier to devise drugs to combat it, and to start developing a vaccine against it. After it had been shown to be a virus of a particular type, scientists had a clear target and were able to make the drugs to combat it. Is the situation similar for non-communicable diseases? To a certain extent, it is. For some cancers, such as those of the liver or cervix, an infectious agent is clearly one of the triggers, so vaccination campaigns should be effective. But such links have not been found for diabetes and cardio-vascular disease, so we have to think again.

We have good ways of treating these diseases once they develop—we know how to lower blood sugar with drugs or insulin, and we can treat high blood pressure and arterial blockages—even if the cost of these treatments puts them beyond the reach of most people in developing countries. But prevention is always better—and cheaper—than treatment. Condoms, safe sex, care about blood transfusions, and avoiding dirty needles are far better strategies for dealing with HIV-AIDS than the expensive triple drug therapy now developed.

So what about diabetes and cardiovascular disease—how can we prevent them? On the face of it the villain causing the problem does not seem hard to find—it is obesity. But, as we will see, while obesity is an important factor, for many people it is not the real culprit, and the plot is not that simple.

Obesity is not just about being a bit fatter, needing to wear a larger size in clothes, and not being able to skip up a flight of stairs. It is not just about the need for wider aeroplane seats or stronger seats on toilets or relabelling the sizes on women's clothes—although a size 12 is not what is used to be. Obesity has major health effects in *raising the risk* of diabetes, heart disease, stroke, asthma, depression, and some forms of cancer. But does it *cause* these diseases? Most doctors and medical scientists, asked to give an instant answer to this question, would say 'Of course it does.' But when we, and they, pause for thought it becomes apparent that the answer is not that simple. We realize that, while there is no doubt that obesity increases the risk of non-communicable disease, it is also clear that it does not cause such disease *directly*. After all, many relatively obese people are as fit as a fiddle. And there are literally millions of relatively young people in, for example, India who have diabetes but who don't appear to be overweight by North American or European standards. So it must be more complicated than just being 'fat'. There must be some other villains missing from the story, some enemies we have not recognized. Tracing those hidden enemies is partly what this book is about.

In a surprisingly short space of time the United Nations, govern-ments, departments of health, doctors, teachers, economists, and the media have become alarmed about obesity. Many young people are quite rightly very worried by it too—for them the publicity about the risks of diabetes and cardiovascular disease associated with obes-ity is as frightening as that about HIV-AIDS was for adolescents of the previous generation. But while it might seem obvious that the problem would be solved if everyone ate less and exercised more, the solution has turned out not to be so simple. We all know that losing weight is hard and keeping it off is even harder. One of the authors has lost more than 20 kg on three separate occasions and, despite his motivation and a career devoted to the issue, has put it back on within months each time!

Losing the obesity war

It is now clear that current and very intensive attempts to tackle the problem of non-communicable disease by aiming to reduce obesity are not working in general. The sad reality is that the global burden of diabe-tes and cardiovascular disease is getting worse. We are losing this war.

The rates of diabetes and cardiovascular disease are high in Western countries, which have well-designed public health systems, despite the enormous efforts of many agencies to make people lose weight. And now these very diseases are also appearing in epidemic fashion in countries far less wealthy—and where most people are not fat by Western standards—such as India, China, and Brazil.

When a proposed solution to a problem fails, there are two possibilities—either the solution is wrong or something is missing in our understanding of the problem. We think that both of these explanations underlie our failure to cope with the global problem of diabetes and cardiovascular disease. We believe that there is a collective misunderstanding of the nature of what is going on and how to address it. But, in addition, could it be that the war is being lost because we are aiming at the wrong target?

Whatever the answer to this question, it seems clear that at best our strategy has been too naive, largely based as it is on attacking a single target—adult obesity. We think that this has come about because those concerned with addressing the problem, from scientists and doctors to health policy makers and funding agencies, have ignored some of the fundamental science. They appear to have been biased towards a particular view of the solution—largely based on the idea that obesity arises from the biblical sins of 'gluttony' and 'sloth' and that diabetes and cardiovascular disease are the inevitable consequences. Then, in the face of evidence that their solution to the problem is not working, they have become even more zealous in their attempts to deal with these two sins and to attack the same target even harder—as if they wore blinkers to prevent them looking for others. A good general would be considering at this point whether there are other ways to win the war. This book aims to remove these biases and to take the blinkers off—before it is too late.

Obesity has been the focus of many public health initiatives. But just because it is a risk factor for diabetes, cardiovascular disease, and some forms of cancer does not mean that it is a disease in itself.

Laying down fat in our bodies is part of normal human biology and we do it from the beginning of our lives, even before we are born. How this fat deposition is controlled, and when it may become a disadvantage, is a subject that we will explore. But we must get away from the 'obesity equals disease' mindset if we are to concentrate less on treating the symptoms and more on preventing the diseases. Many health professionals and organizations focus on interventions in the increasing number of people who are obese. While this is undoubtedly important, we will see that it is as urgent to focus on the pathways that lead children to *become* obese.

The rise in the incidence of diabetes and cardiovascular disease in India, China, parts of South-East Asia (especially Malaysia and Indonesia), the Middle East, and South America has occurred within a generation. The speed of this effect is alarming and the implications are enormous. Already 100 million people in China and perhaps even more in India now have diabetes. Cardiovascular disease, manifest as stroke, high blood pressure, heart attack, or heart failure, is also rife. The rate of diabetes in the Middle East and North Africa is almost incomprehensible—over 20 per cent of people in the United Arab Emirates now have diabetes and there is no sign that this number is falling. More than 70 per cent of adults and 22 per cent of children are overweight in this region. Similar figures for diabetes exist for Colombo in Sri Lanka. The statistics for small Pacific states like Nauru and Tonga exceed even these numbers.

Worse still, we are now starting to see the same thing happening in sub-Saharan Africa, in societies which have only just begun to climb out of the abyss of poverty. Across the developing world a tragedy is about to be played out with sickening speed, because these countries are almost totally unprepared to deal with such a rapidly rising burden of new disease. They cannot afford to vaccinate every child against infectious diseases such as polio or measles, or to provide antibiotics to treat patients with tuberculosis. They cannot afford mosquito nets for every bed. If they do not have the resources to address the long-standing problems of infectious, or communicable, disease, what hope do they have of tackling diabetes and cardiovascular disease?

The wheel of fortune

At the end of his great tragic play *King Lear*, Shakespeare uses the metaphor of the wheel of fortune to make the fate of his characters even more poignant. Surely when fate has taken them to the depths of misfortune, the wheel cannot take them further down—surely life can only improve? Not so for Lear or, we fear, for the developing world. Things will almost certainly get worse. In developing countries we see diabetes occurring in much younger people than in the past, or than usually occurs in the West. We can only imagine the humanitarian and financial costs of large numbers of people developing such disease in their thirties, when their productive working lives may be drastically shortened and they still have young families to support. In addition they will need drug treatment for decades, and the accumulating costs of this will be horrendous. The wheel of fortune can take many people lower down still.

Why can't we stop this wheel going down? We seem to clutch at it with feeble hands, as if we didn't have the strength. But in reality we do not know *how* to slow it down. Nor do we yet seem to have built up the resolve to tackle the problem or mustered the right forces to do so. Why is this happening—why for example does an Indian or Chinese person not need to be as obese as a white European to suffer from heart disease or diabetes? Why are these diseases appearing at ever younger ages in developed countries and at even younger ages in developing countries? Providing some answers to these questions is central to this book.

Then there is a broader and even more worrying turn of events. The worry is that, beyond causing illness and death and slowing down economic development, diabetes and cardiovascular disease may have geopolitical consequences too. It is obvious that the changing pattern of disease in India, China, and Indonesia is in some way associated with the adoption of aspects of the so-called Western lifestyle—foods high in calories and fat, often of low nutritional quality, lower levels of physical activity, and a number of other changes which we will come back to later. Could it be that, as the economic burden of hundreds of millions of people with diabetes and heart disease and their accompanying complications of strokes, kidney failure, blindness, and limb amputations descends on these developing nations, disabling people still in the prime of their lives and stretching healthcare systems beyond their limits, the West will be blamed for exporting an unhealthy lifestyle to these nations, driven by the profits of globalization? Will this create a new clash of cultures and give rise to a new set of tensions, or something even worse? At the very least it seems likely to damage relations between the developed and developing nations at a time when we need much closer collaboration if we are to address the other global challenges of climate change, fossil fuel use, water and food security, and terrorism.

As we have changed the way we live and what we eat, the incidence of obesity, diabetes, and cardiovascular disease has increased dramatically. The changes in the way we live are a direct result of many advances in technology, the nature of the food we eat, and the way we conduct our lives. Humans now live longer and healthier lives than ever before in our evolutionary history. Yet the irony is that the very technological advances that allow us to have these longer lives may now compromise the way we live them. There can be no doubt that changes in lifestyle are fundamental to the problems of obesity, diabetes, and cardiovascular disease, and we strongly believe in the importance of healthy eating, exercise, and avoidance of tobacco products. Nothing in this book is meant to undermine that message. But these measures in themselves, while necessary, will not be sufficient to slow the relentless downward lurch of the wheel of fortune.

Our longer lives are in no small part due to the tremendous improvements in public health over the past two centuries. We have made great strides in developing vaccines, antibiotics, and antiseptic agents to prevent and treat many bacterial diseases, and drugs to combat malaria as well as worm and other parasite infestations. In addition, we have endeavoured to make supplies of clean water available to everyone and to channel our sewage safely away. This has been achieved in the developed world, although there is still much to be done across Africa and other parts of the less developed world.

In the West these improvements in public health and the development of modern medicine can be traced back to the beginning of the industrial revolution, although they gained prominence in the mid 19th and particularly the 20th centuries. But it is really only since the Second World War and the beginning of the end of colonialism that we have seen the same phenomenon happen in much poorer countries. The good news is that many improvements in public health are taking place much more quickly than they did in developed societies. In many developing countries, for example, the so-called nutritional transition—from hunger and famine to food security—is happening over just one generation, rather than over several generations as it did in developed countries.

The nutritional transition

The nutritional transition is not just about the amounts of food available. It is also about its quality. Food security, that is ensuring there is enough food reaching the world's population, is a growing concern but this is largely, although not entirely, beyond the scope of this book. But food security is only part of the nutritional challenge we face. The nutritional transition is really a covert revolution in the way we feed ourselves. It involves a shift from basic unrefined foods such as pulses, grain, fruit and vegetables, fish or lean meat, to highly processed foods. In many places this has happened in a decade or less and everywhere it has had undesirable biological effects on our bodies through new challenges, which our bodies cannot always handle.

Because of this nutritional transition there has been a marked change in our daily intake of high-calorie, sugary, and fatty foods. The food revolution has been given further impetus by sophisticated marketing and by the shift to fast or convenience foods associated with other lifestyle changes. This nutritional change has been played out against the background of apparently much lower physical energy expenditure as the burden of manual labour decreases and we move to mechanized transport and favour electronic entertainment over physical activities and sports for recreation.

Flagging up these changes is not a novel idea—so why are we doing it? Because of the widespread supposition that, as the modern diet and our lower level of daily physical exercise exacerbate the risk of obesity, *therefore* the best approach for addressing the problem must be to target diet or exercise, especially in people who are already obese. We believe that there are fundamental flaws in this argument and that more comprehensive and holistic approaches are urgently needed.

This dominant public health message, urging dietary restraint and more exercise, is part of a set of strongly held beliefs among many doctors and public health specialists. We say 'beliefs' in the plural, because there is no agreement on a single effective strategy for reducing obesity. There has been a debate between the experts who claim that tackling it is primarily about promoting exercise, and those who claim that it is all about diet, a particular kind of diet, or avoiding certain food components such as trans-fats or omega-6 fatty acids. But as yet no one has come up with the magic bullet intervention which works infallibly to reduce obesity. We do not think that this bullet will ever be found because, while the goal is laudable, these approaches are oversimplified and, unfortunately, are based on incomplete knowledge of human biology. We don't seem to be willing to look more broadly at the scientific evidence. Beware the expert who claims that a complex problem has a simple answer.

We know that the problem we face is associated with our modern lifestyle, even if it is not simply caused by it. So is the solution just to return to a traditional pre-industrial lifestyle? Maybe in theory, but unfortunately this is not realistic—even though many books have been written on the benefits of the hunter-gatherer or Palaeolithic diet, and so on. The majority of these represent folksy science rather than objective and reliable knowledge. They are effectively meaningless. It is no more feasible for the majority of the world's population to move back to such a lifestyle than it would be to propose living in today's world without the internet.

This is not to say that we should not encourage healthier eating and more walking, cycling, and exercise in general, which like stopping smoking, have health benefits at any age. Indeed we are strong advocates for the value of such measures. But, equally, we have to realize that there is a limit to what can be achieved through such initiatives, and to the benefits which we can expect from such an approach. To achieve more—and we absolutely have to achieve more—we have to take a different, more sophisticated, and more scientific approach.

Governing bodies

What we have just said could be seen as heresy. The relationship of obesity with diabetes, cardiovascular disease, and other non-communicable diseases is well recognized and we do not dispute the general association. In the main the thinner people are, the healthier they will be. However, governments, the World Health Organization, and other agencies have focused their attention almost entirely on smoking and obesity for the past decade. The battle against tobacco is being won, at least in developed if not in developing countries. But despite the millions of dollars spent, the obesity strategy is not working—the incidence of obesity and chronic disease is rising in every country, from rich to poor. We have been dismayed, and not a little angered, that this approach to the problem—eat less high-energy food and exercise more—seems to have remained unchanged even though it has not delivered the hoped-for benefits. Quite simply, people are getting fatter.

The sad reality is that for a great many people diet and exercise just do not work, at least over the long term. Many people try hard to diet, but find it tougher than fighting well-recognized addictions such as smoking. This in itself raises the question: can eating itself be an addiction? There is evidence that for some people it really is, although, as we will see, there may be different underlying biological mechanisms. But even if a person is able to curb their appetite and stick with one of the myriad popularized diets which are pushed at them—the Atkins diet, the grapefruit diet, the low-carb diet, the low-fat diet, and so forth—they may lose weight initially but many cannot keep that weight off. Then again, some people find taking more exercise easy while others find it hard to sustain. Some succeed in beating obesity, but many others do not. Should we be surprised by this? Hardly—just as in other aspects of our lives, we are all different and our biology is designed to make it hard to lose weight.

Such differences are the stuff of anecdotes in almost every family—the great aunt who had an enormous appetite yet was as thin as a twig all her life, and the uncle who starved himself but could still never buy trousers wide enough to fit him. There are people who are fat but do not suffer from disease, while others suffer from diabetes and/or heart disease but do not appear to be very fat. These simple observations about our biological differences are a fundamental theme which runs through this book. We will explain some aspects of human biology which probably won't surprise many non-scientists—because they are reminiscent of those family stories—but which somehow seem to have eluded the attention of the specialists in this field. People are different—some people appear to be at greater risk of ill health than others even if they exercise and eat the same diet. This is true in every society even if some societies seem more at risk than others.

That non-communicable diseases have become a critical issue for the world community is now indisputable. In September 2011, while this book was in press, the United Nations General Assembly held a special Summit devoted to non-communicable disease prevention and treatment, especially in developing countries. During the planning stages there was little indication that its focus would shift much from the traditional view narrowly focused on adult lifestyle. We felt that too many policy makers and their advisers still wear blinkers when it comes to seeing what to do and how to go about doing it.

But we are not saying that everything should be left to governments and the organizations that represent them, such as the United Nations. There are other important and influential non-government organizations that can play a major role, and some of these have more funds to deploy than many governments. An example is the Bill and Melinda Gates Foundation. So far, the Gates Foundation has largely been engaged in the prevention of communicable disease. It has provided millions of dollars for research on new technologies such as developing vaccines to fight malaria and HIV-AIDS. So far it has scarcely turned its attention to non-communicable diseases—and this is revealing.

The Gates Foundation would acknowledge that for infectious diseases vaccines are only part of the answer. Fighting malaria requires a range of coordinated approaches—draining swamps, providing chemically treated mosquito nets, developing new drugs for those who have caught resistant strains of malaria to stop the transmission of these strains, and so on. Combating HIV-AIDS similarly requires education about drugs and safe sex, access to condoms or other barrier contraceptives, and advanced drug therapies. A vaccine is not yet on the horizon despite years of work because this is difficult science—the biology of the HIV virus is such that a vaccine is hard to devise, hard to develop, and hard to test. And so the Gates Foundation and others have had the insight to shift to a much more multidimensional approach to communicable disease. We need to take a similar approach to fighting non-communicable disease and we need the charitable and philanthropic sector to realize that this merits as much attention as infectious disease, even though it is apparently less dramatic and less easily fixed.

First steps towards disease

If battling infectious disease is complicated, battling diabetes and cardiovascular disease is proving to be even more complex. Until recently it was hoped that discoveries of genetic differences would explain the variation in disease risk which we find between individuals. However, while variation in our genes accounts for some of our differences in risk, it is not as much as we had previously hoped, or as advocates of genetic medicine had prophesied. Not only is the effect of our genes on our risks of obesity, diabetes, and cardiovascular disease small, but it does not easily explain the patterns of obesity and non-communicable disease that we observe around the world.

Besides, if the problem lay solely in our genes we would have little capacity beyond the implausible use of gene therapy to change our fate. This would be a depressing scenario. But fortunately there is much more to health and disease than our genes. Nonetheless, if individual variation in the settings of our appetites and our metabolic controls can be explained at least in part by genetic variation, we might, through genetic research, get some clues to the complex processes by which diabetes and cardiovascular disease develop. And indeed such science is finding new and exciting explanations that do offer hope for intervention.

We now recognize that even some children and young people who are not obviously fat may already be on a path to diabetes and cardiovascular disease later in their lives, and that it is not easy to switch them to a healthier path. In the last two decades there has been an explosion of knowledge which shows that what happens even before we are born can put us on the path to obesity and risk of non-communicable disease.

We will explain in the second half of this book that there are several developmental paths to obesity and to diabetes and cardiovascular disease, and that obesity and disease risk are starting to appear in childhood more and more. A woman who is obese may have children who are more likely to become obese; the incidence of diabetes in pregnancy is rising, and the effects of this on the fetus can lead to a higher risk of obesity and diabetes in the next generation. Babies who are born prematurely or small are at greater risk; twins, which are increasingly common in a world where women have their babies later and where the need for techniques such as in-vitro fertilization is becoming common, are at greater risk. And fathers may have something to do with it as well. There is much to think about here.

Perhaps from this list we can begin to see how important it is to understand the fundamental biology of how risk is set up during our individual development as fetus and infant. We do not leave this part of our lives behind when we are born or when we are weaned. We carry all this biological history, unremembered, around with us for the rest of our lives. No wonder that we all differ as adults in our risk of obesity and in our responses—or lack of responses—to simple interventions such as dieting or exercise. No wonder that this leads to differences in our risk of diabetes and cardiovascular disease.

It used to be thought that most of these developmental risks could be captured in the measurement of birth weight, because this seemed to indicate how well the mother's womb had provided the resources needed for the baby to grow to his or her genetic potential. As research has progressed, however, we find that many much more subtle influences on fetal development, which are not reflected in changes in birth weight, also affect later disease patterns. Many of these influences reflect the mother's nutrition or health, often even before she became pregnant. Sometimes they even depend on the health of *her* mother. They may be affected by the health and lifestyle of the father too. We will explore this very important new research in this book because it leads us to the conclusion that a very high percentage of us have echoes of developmental factors in our bodies which play a major role in our later risk of ill health.

These developmental influences may appear subtle, but they are also commonplace. One somewhat surprising but important example is that recent research shows that first-born children are at greater risk of developing obesity than subsequent children of the same woman. Think of the questions which this observation, which is statistically robust, raises. Should women have different diets before or during their first pregnancy? Should we treat first-born children differently to reduce their risk? What are the socio-economic implications of this in urban China, where legislation has restricted family size to one child?

Such descriptive observations are all very well but they may not actually be very helpful if we do not know the underlying biology— in other words, what is cause and what is effect. Increasingly, however, we are gaining insights into how such effects work, and we realize that they are part of fundamental biological processes which many other species use in their development too. Those who work in this field are convinced that here lies an important missing link in the problem of variation between people in risk of obesity, diabetes, and cardiovascular disease. This new knowledge may help us to mount an effective set of strategies to address the problem.

Blinkered

There is a large body of scientific evidence for these ideas, yet somehow we feel that we are being controversial in voicing them.

The developmental perspective on diabetes and cardiovascular disease appears to go against the grain of current wisdom in this area. We can see this from a very recent example. In October 2010 the Organisation for Economic Co-operation and Development, the intergovernmental think tank of advanced nations on economic issues, produced a report on obesity. It runs to many pages, and was the culmination of years of work. Yet despite its apparent sophistication, it failed to mention development once, despite the overwhelming scientific evidence for its importance. Nor did it discuss the problems of inadequate or excessive weight gain, obesity, or diabetes in pregnancy. Although we single this report out for example, it is typical of a body of work and a tradition in public health. The blinkers seem to fit very comfortably, it seems. Why?

The practicalities of modern science and policy formation provide an explanation in part. The methods for studying risk factors in populations of adults are often limited by allowing us to look only at current factors such as smoking, diet, and exercise. They do not let us look backwards from adulthood into early life readily, if at all. The research needed to do this takes many years and is expensive. It is perhaps not surprising that it has taken time for a sufficient body of knowledge to be built up to demonstrate the importance of early development. But now that we have such knowledge, there is no excuse for ignoring its implications any longer.

There are vested interests as well as these down-to-earth practicalities which have hindered progress here too. Some drug companies would much rather focus on treating disease than preventing it, especially if prevention has to start in childhood when drug therapy is undesirable. Much of the food industry focuses on the profits to be made from fast foods and energy-dense fatty and sweet foods and drinks. Politicians and the electorate would, understandably, rather focus on the here and now than see their tax revenue directed towards interventions to prevent disease likely to occur more than ten years later.

Unfortunately, if we ignore the developmental perspective, we may miss the biggest opportunity for effective intervention. Indeed, a recent UK government think tank, the Obesity Taskforce of the Foresight Group, identified development in early life as the only time when effective strategies to deal with the problem of obesity are likely to be successful. And we have some pretty good ideas of strategies—some practical, some still on the horizon—which give us hope.

But to get to the point of actually implementing these strategies means thinking beyond our biases and taking our blinkers off.

And here we meet other cultural and social factors in operation. In Western countries those of lowest socio-economic status are most at risk. Is this simply because poorer people buy cheaper food, which is often of lower nutritional quality, or are there more complex factors operating? We will have to discuss this in this book. Moreover, there are big cultural differences in how people perceive their body shapes. So, when we try to reduce obesity in a population, are we addressing concepts of body shape or the wish to prevent disease? Certainly, for most people in developed countries it is the former—after all, the diet industry is built upon images of glamour and sexuality, not on preventing disease. We need to consider the implications of this too.

We wrote this book with two goals in mind. First, we wanted to show that the problem of obesity and the all too common non-communicable diseases actually looks different if we take off our blinkers—suddenly we see that we need to do more than talk about diet and exercise, bemoaning the shortcomings of people for whom these do not work. And we see that new scientific discoveries about human development give new insights into why the incidence of diabetes and cardiovascular disease is increasing, and novel ways of detecting early in their lives the people who will be most at risk later.

Our second goal is to lay down a challenge—especially to governments, to NGOs, and to many agencies—to think outside the box, to take a more holistic view which extends beyond entrenched biases.

They need to consider the enormous social and cultural variations that limit personal motivations. They need to understand that the issue is not simply about choosing to be slothful and gluttonous. They need to understand that a healthy world starts with healthy parents, which leads to healthy fetuses, healthy infants, healthy children, healthy adolescents, and then to healthy adults.

We will argue that until such a life-course perspective, along with a deeper understanding of why people live their lives in the ways that they do, has been incorporated into policy we will not change substantially the fate of many of us around the world. We will be destined to get fatter and more of us will suffer from disease.

2

Fat Chances

Why are we so worked up about fat?

If we live in a developed country where the average income is high, it is impossible to ignore the collective and entirely justifiable hysteria about fat. There is story after story about how our population is getting more obese. And this does not apply just to adults, for children and even infants are becoming obese too. Governments are being urged to tackle the problem, to give it a much greater priority, because the human cost of obesity is enormous.

Take a walk on the Bund in Shanghai or in the Zócalo in Mexico City. You come across well-dressed young children being walked to a museum by their teachers. The children are lively, animated, and excited, but one thing stands out—they look increasingly like children in London or Chicago or Sydney—many of them are plump. Sit in a cafe in a provincial town such as Arequipa in Peru, or in Udaipur in India, and again you will see many young adults who look on the fat side. Does this really matter? Isn't it just a matter of aesthetics? We live in today's world, and today humans tend to be fat. Shouldn't we just stop worrying about it?

No.

Excess fat, depending where it is in the body, is a major risk factor for disease. The lifespan of someone who is obese (with a body mass index or BMI of 40–45) is eight to ten years shorter than that of someone who is not. The effects are graded, getting worse as fat builds up in our bodies. Someone of average height who is overweight will increase their risk of death by about 30 per cent for every 15 kg of excess weight they carry. The chances of disability—from whatever cause—are twice as great in people who are obese as in those who are not.

Adult onset diabetes, heart disease, high blood pressure, and stroke are all much more likely if we are obese. The same is true of joint disease, kidney and reproductive problems, and even some mental illnesses. Most people in the world will die from one of these non-communicable diseases, and because their detrimental effects start well before death occurs, their impact on both an individual's life and their ability to contribute to society is enormous. The cost to the health sector and to the broader economy of a nation is almost immeasurable. Most attempts to put a price on the problem are horrifying, but are almost certainly underestimations. The World Economic Forum recently calculated that non-communicable disease will cost the world more than US$50 trillion over the next ten years.

These diseases are now as much of a problem in the developing world as in the developed world. And as people in the developing world live longer when other aspects of their lives improve, the rate will rise even more. And there is now evidence that being obese is a risk factor for some cancers of the breast, colon, and perhaps the uterus, oesophagus, and kidney. It has been calculated that 25 per cent of premature deaths of women over the age of 50 in the United States would be prevented every year if they were not so fat.

But we have to be careful about how we interpret such figures. Obesity on a global scale itself was rarely a health problem in its own right until recently. We see television stories about 300-pound people suffering from morbid obesity who cannot move from their homes, who cannot breathe properly, and whose skeletons cannot support their weight. These are real problems and often there is an underlying medical explanation for this extreme obesity. But increasingly, we also tend to stigmatize fat people and people with relatively lower degrees of obesity. This does not help, of course, for it can affect their mental health and, paradoxically, increase their obesity.

But morbid obesity is not the prime focus of this book. In relation to the magnitude of the chronic disease problem, it is still small. We will focus on the issues of diabetes and cardiovascular disease and their relationship to much lower degrees of obesity. Too many people in every country on the planet are being affected, or will be affected, by these diseases. What is worrying is that these diseases are striking at much younger ages. Thirty years ago a child with type 2 diabetes was a medical rarity—now in Western countries more than half the children attending a diabetes clinic suffer from type 2 diabetes.

So we need to ask the right question: how can we reduce the burden of non-communicable disease? It is only within the framework of this more direct question that obesity becomes relevant. Not all fat is necessarily bad. For example, steatopygia—the technical name given to the large fat stores on the buttocks which are particularly prominent in peoples of sub-Saharan African origin—is a big fat deposit but it does not do any harm. There is no evidence that having steatopygia affects the risk of disease. Indeed it is thought to be a special adaptation which evolved to allow humans to live in unpredictable environments by storing energy in the form of fat for periods when food was not plentiful. We need to see beyond fat itself to understand why it is that excess fat in some parts of the body and in some people is not good.

What fat does

Fat is complicated stuff. Of all the components of the human body it is the one which varies most between individuals. It is generally considered healthy to have about 15 per cent of one's body made up of fat if one is male and about 20 per cent if female, although some of us have less than that. This proportion of fat, about one-sixth of the body, is probably about the same as that of our ancestors in the Rift Valley in Africa in the early stages of human evolution.

For many years we have viewed fat simply as a storage depot, a source of spare energy which we carry around with us, rather in the way that we might take a snack or even a packed meal on a long journey. As a species we do not graze more or less continuously while we are awake, unlike many large vegetarian mammals. Rather, we eat substantial meals at intervals and can then go for many hours—for example when we sleep—or even days in between.

Fat is different from protein and carbohydrate, not only in its chemical structure but also in the amount of energy it stores. This is important because the body uses energy to run all its machinery. This energy is generated by organelles within cells called mitochondria which use oxygen carried by the bloodstream to burn the fuel supplies available to them. This is very similar to a stove which creates energy in the form of heat by using oxygen from the air to burn wood or coal or natural gas. And just as these fuels generate very different amounts of heat, so is fat different from the other possible body fuels. One gram of fat produces 9 calories, more than twice the amount of energy produced by burning protein or carbohydrates. This is why fat is the energy store of choice for a camel, a migrating bird or insect, or any other animal that faces long periods without access to food as part of its life.

We not only eat fat and store that fat in our bodies, but if we have excess energy intake from other sources, we can also convert carbohydrates, particularly alcohol and sugars, and even protein indirectly into fat. So any form of energy we consume can, under some circumstances, end up as fat.

Life is all about energy—without it we are dead. Everything our bodies do requires energy—our brains use a lot of it; so do the heart as it pumps blood and our intestines as they digest and absorb food. Every aspect of body function is energy-dependent. Then of course we use energy to keep warm and when we move our muscles as we walk or run, when we stand, even when we fidget. Different forms of exercise and activity consume different amounts of calories (or kilo-joules, which is another measure of energy; 4 kilojoules equal about 1 calorie). Growth also requires energy to convert food into new body tissues—and reproduction shifts fuel supplies to the fetus as we build the next generation.

So, when we look at fat we see that it is not an inert, static part of our bodies like the snack we might carry in a pocket. The fat stored is the result of the balance between 'energy in' in the form of food and 'energy out' in the form of our normal body functions and of growth, reproduction, and exercise. Essentially the only way we have to store excess energy is in the form of fat, so if we eat more energy than we expend there is only one way in which that excess energy can be stored, and that is as fat. Similarly, if we expend more energy than we consume, we usually lose fat. There are exceptions which can lead to muscle and protein loss but these are associated with disease such as cancer.

We all need some fat in our bodies—we would not survive without it. Indeed when we are born we are the fattest species on the planet—human babies at birth are fatter even than baby seals or whales. For many years it was assumed that we evolved to have fat babies because fat, as a good insulator, keeps babies warm—this is why adult polar mammals like whales and seals have so much blubber. But we now know that this is not likely to be the reason—after all, our ancestors were born into hot climates in Africa. Our exceptional fatness at birth is probably due to the newborn baby's development being dependent on having spare energy to protect its very energy-dependent brain growth, particularly if its energy intake becomes limited by illnesses such as diarrhoea. Such illnesses were historically very common around the time of weaning when the infant starts to consume a range of new foods. Unlike its mother's breast milk, which is virtually sterile, these new foods contain all sorts of pathogenic organisms. These diseases are still very common in the developing world where diarrhoea remains a major cause of infant death—and death is far more likely if the baby is chronically under-nourished and has inadequate fat stores.

Until recently much of the focus of obesity research has been based on the concept of the energy balance equation, namely that the amount of fat you have is the outcome of the balance between energy taken in as food and energy expended by muscular activity, maintaining the body, and even thinking. So some people store more fat either because they have eaten more over a sustained period of time or because they have expended less energy over that period of time. The only way to change the amount of fat in their bodies is for them to eat less or to expend more energy. There is truth in this idea, but only some. It is certainly true that we can lose weight by taking up an active sport or adopting a daily exercise regime. Marathon runners and even habitual joggers are often fairly thin. But then they often eat substantial meals and indulge in snacks too. So it is not just that they have burnt off more fat, because they seem to be taking on board more energy as well. It is almost as if the throughput of energy, from food taken in to energy output, has been increased, like a car with a slipping clutch that uses a lot of fuel to go any distance.

Equally, many of us know how difficult it is to lose fat by dieting. Limiting how much we eat will usually lead to some loss of weight, but very often we put it back on again even though we maintain a strict diet. No matter how determined the slimmer becomes in terms of restricting his or her calorie intake, somehow the body just seems to become more efficient at fuel usage and at keeping up the body's fat stores. Indeed we are now finding that there is some very complex brain and hormonal biology that tries to restore our weight to what it was originally. That is why few people can sustain weight loss over many years.

The fat controller

This brings us to the idea that we all have a set point for regulating the level of our body fat. It is not simply that any calories ingested and not burnt in energy expenditure are stashed away as fat globules. It appears that the level of fat in our bodies is carefully controlled from day to day and from year to year throughout our lives. The control sets how much and what we eat, how much energy we are willing to expend in physical exercise, how we control our body temperature, and even how much energy we waste everyday by fidgeting or save when we are inactive or asleep. These processes are underpinned by some fundamental aspects of our biology.

Fat is not just like the balance of money in a bank account at the end of the month, when we try to weigh up how much we have spent against how much we have earned. That balance is controlled by how profligate or abstemious we have been in the month and maybe how much our employer has deigned to pay us. The balance is the result of the operation of the two opposing processes of spending and being paid, something which control engineers call an 'emergent property' of the system. But with fat it is the very level in the body itself which is controlled. The financial analogy would be that we must retain £1,000 in our bank account at all times, so we then regulate our expenditure or our earnings in order to maintain that balance on a day-to-day basis. Here the engineer would say that it's the spending or the taking on of more or less employment in order to maintain the £1,000 balance which forms the emergent properties of the system.

But how is the level of fat in the body controlled? Or, to put it another way, how does the body know how much fat it has? The bank account analogy doesn't help very much here, because, after all, you can use your debit card to buy a new pair of shoes for £50 just as easily if you have £100 in your account as if you have £1,000 in your account. And equally, you can deposit money into your account just as easily no matter what the balance is. The regulation of spending or earning is not directly related to whether we set our desired minimal balance at £1,000 or £10. We can regulate that balance only by taking a reading of it, say from the internet or a cash machine. So the body must have a sensor, some means of detecting how much fat is stored, which must somehow interact with the systems which regulate how much fat there is.

But fat is not just a passive storage system like the gas tank in a car or your bank account. Research over the last 20 or so years has shown that fat produces a range of hormones which affect the ways our body works. The most well-known hormone made by fat cells is called leptin. Leptin enters the bloodstream, and when it reaches the brain it affects appetite. High levels of leptin suppress appetite and give us a sense of being satiated. Leptin can also affect other organs; for example the pancreas, where it alters the amount of insulin made to control blood sugar. There are other hormones which also affect our appetite control, some of them made by the stomach in response to food, of which the most important is called ghrelin. When the stomach is not full it secretes ghrelin, which stimulates our appetite—so we start looking for food.

The importance of the satiety hormone leptin can be seen from observations on children who have a genetic defect which prevents them from producing a functional form of the hormone, or whose appetite and satiety control centres in the brain are resistant to it. A team in Cambridge led by the ebullient and talented scientist Steve O'Rahilly, who is both a clinician and a molecular geneticist, have studied such children. They are exceptionally obese. They are almost unable to move around and certainly not able to join their friends in playing sport, dancing, or riding a bicycle. They are driven by an insatiable appetite, to the point where they absolutely have to eat. Some of them have been known to raid the freezer in the middle of the night to eat uncooked frozen food to satisfy this craving. Steve and his group are adamant that these children are not just greedy, and there is very little that they can do about the problem themselves. Nor is it simply like a drug addiction. It is not just because they have developed a taste for ice cream and chocolate sauce and have a habit they cannot break. The setting of their appetite control is fundamentally wrong. But for those rare few who have a genetic defect that hinders their production of functional leptin, treating them with doses of synthetic leptin hormone can help them to lose huge amounts of weight and restore their lives to some semblance of normality.

And when we lose weight, our plasma ghrelin levels tend to rise and our leptin levels fall. These two hormonal changes act on our brains to make us eat more and return to our original weights. These changes can be seen even years after weight loss. This makes sustaining weight loss very difficult.

But not all fat is the same. From the perspective of metabolic disease the most important fat is not the fat directly under our skin, at least that fat under the skin on our arms and legs and back, although there is an exception which we will soon discuss. This fat seems quieter in a hormonal sense—some experts have argued that it simply provides a way of storing energy and, unless it contributes to morbid obesity and interferes with breathing and weight-bearing, it is not harmful. Fat is also stored in breast tissue in women because healthy pregnancies and lactation require an adequate energy store, as reflected in adequate fat stores. Sexual selection theory in evolution would also suggest that males choose their mates partly on the basis of their breasts because this aspect of the body's shape can represent fertility.

Instead it is the fat deeper inside our bodies that really plays a major role in influencing whether we are healthy or not. This is the fat we cannot see. It is normally found lining the inside of the abdomen and in the membranes supporting the intestines. Technically this is called visceral fat. This fat is metabolically very easy to mobilize and indeed we use it to provide energy to deal with short-term fasting for a day or so. This can happen if we are ill but it might have been very common for our hunter-gatherer ancestors at times when no food could be found. Visceral fat also has very different biological functions from fat under the skin because it makes different hormones and inflammatory compounds. As our fat stores increase, we deposit excess amounts of this internal fat, not only in the intestinal membranes but also inside our livers and even inside our blood vessels and hearts. This is not healthy and is associated with a change in the way these organs work and how they respond to insulin. When this happens we are on the path to diabetes and cardiovascular disease.

But it turns out that some fat deep under our skin on the abdomen is biochemically very similar to visceral fat. Thus unhealthy obesity is generally associated with increases in fat both inside and outside the abdomen. That is why having obesity centred on the abdomen is a particular risk factor, and we can assess it by measuring the ratio of waist to hip circumferences, or simply our waist circumference.

The foods we eat contain very many different kinds of fat— unsaturated or saturated fats, omega-3 or omega-6 fats, and so on. These different names refer to the biochemical structure of fat. The simplest form of fat consists essentially of a long chain of carbon atoms joined together with hydrogen and oxygen molecules attached. But not all fats are these simple lipids; some are joined to glycerol to form what are called triglycerides, which are made of a glycerol molecule attached to three fat molecules. Fats travel in the bloodstream from the liver, where they are first received after digestion or are made from other food types, to fat tissue. Or they can travel back to liver and muscle for burning. When fats travel in the bloodstream they are attached to proteins called lipoproteins. It is the different levels of triglycerides and lipoproteins in a blood sample that doctors use to assess our fat status and one of the risk factors for disease.

Cholesterol is also biochemically related to fat and is often found in food in association with fats. Its structure consists of a set of rings made of carbon atoms. It is a much more complex molecule for our bodies to make, but the liver can produce it. We need cholesterol to make steroid hormones and for some other building blocks of our bodies. But we also consume cholesterol in our diet and, like its linear cousins, it can get deposited in our blood vessels and damage their functions or even block them. Blocked blood vessels in the brain cause strokes and in the heart they cause a heart attack.

There is increasing evidence that what we eat can change our body's fat composition. For example, women who eat a lot of food containing omega-6 fats produce breast milk which has higher concentrations of omega-6 fats. Human milk, like animal milk, is fat-rich because this is the best way of providing the energy that the growing baby needs. Over the past 20 years the ratio of omega-6 to omega-3 fatty acids in human milk has doubled, reflecting the much higher intakes of omega-6 fatty acids in the modern Western diet. The biggest source of omega-6 fatty acids comes from cereal grains whereas omega-3 fatty acids are found in the highest concentration in fish oil. Similarly, depending on how much cholesterol we consume, we can change its levels in our blood. But because we also make cholesterol in our liver, people with dangerously high levels of cholesterol need to take drugs such as statins to reduce the risk of blood vessel damage.

White or brown

Our focus so far has been on what we call white fat—this is the fat we are worried about because it is associated with the risk of cardiovascular disease and diabetes. But there is another kind, called brown fat. Newborn babies have much more of this fat than adults. It is found around the kidneys, between the shoulder blades, and at the base of the neck. Even though adults have less brown fat, we may be able to increase the amount we have—for example, there is some evidence that exposure to cold can induce more to form.

Why is some fat brown, and why is this medically good fat? The colour difference is due to the fact that it contains many more mitochondria, the energy-producing factories of the cell. Mitochondria throughout the body generate the energy for the cells to work by burning fuels including fat. But we also need to generate heat, because we are a warm-blooded species and our biology is designed to work at a body temperature of 37 °C. That is the temperature at which our enzymes and body function have been optimized over evolutionary time. If our body temperature is too cold we do not cope well—death from hypothermia will occur if we cannot warm up. And we all know how awful we feel if we have a temperature which is too high. Heat is just a form of energy and all our cells contribute to generating it to keep us at 37 °C. But brown fat is particularly good at generating heat and that is why newborn babies have much more of it. One of the most important transitions from being a fetus to being a baby is to start controlling body temperature. Premature babies are much less efficient at maintaining their body temperature because they have less brown fat. For this reason we may have to keep them warm in an incubator to survive. Strangely, the incubator was first developed for showing off premature babies in sideshows, like circus freaks at the St Louis World's Fair in 1904.

Brown fat produces more heat than white fat because its mitochondria have different settings. So rather than storing energy, these mitochondria produce heat. This is called 'uncoupling' and has been known in principle for many years, although its biochemical pathways in the mitochondria have only been described in detail in the past two decades.

One of the first observations of the function of brown fat arose during the First World War in women working in munitions factories in France. They were packing explosives into the shells used to bombard German trenches so futilely and tragically in the Somme. The women were observed to be taking rather too much time off work. True, the conditions in the factories were fairly bad by today's standards but there was a war on and Lord Kitchener's finger, pointing directly at the viewer from behind his handlebar moustache on thousands of posters, made it clear that every citizen was expected to do his or her duty.

These factory workers said that they felt pretty sick and found it hard to come in to work. Some of them would start a day's work but have to go home early. Were they really ill or just malingering? It seemed that they were ill because they certainly had high temperatures. Perhaps the crowded conditions of the factories were conducive to the spread of some infection. But if it was truly an infection, it was very nasty indeed and one that had not previously been encountered in medicine. Some workers developed temperatures which rose very rapidly during the day; they sweated profusely and began to shiver, and had to be taken to the sick room where colleagues covered them with blankets in the hope of stopping their shivering. But their temperature rose still higher and several of them died.

Clearly this situation could not be allowed to continue, for the sake of the war effort if not for the health of the munitions factory workers. Observation of the patterns of illness, associated as they were with the working day and only occurring in some workers in the factory, finally led to the answer. The workers were being continually exposed to the substance dinitrophenol, a key ingredient of the explosives packed into the shells. Dinitrophenol changes the biochemistry of mitochondria so that even those in white fat start burning fuel like brown fat—it uncouples mitochondrial metabolism so that energy is produced as heat rather than as metabolic energy.

What has fat got to do with disease?

We have already said that, except in cases of gross obesity such as those caused by genetic defects, simply being fat in itself does not directly cause disease. But being fat changes our risk of getting disease. And it does so in several ways—some direct and some indirect.

While fats are essential to our body function and some are essential in our diet, excessive intakes of cholesterol and of some specific forms of fat are more likely to be harmful. For example infant milks are supplemented with the unsaturated omega-3 fat called DHA because we believe this is essential for brain development—indeed the brain depends on many special fats to function properly, and DHA is a type of fat which our bodies cannot efficiently make from other fats. But other fats may not be so healthy. Saturated fats are not as healthy as unsaturated fats. The membranes of cells are made from fatty molecules and if the diet is high in the wrong kind of fats the cell membrane composition changes and this in turn alters the way the cells function.

As our body levels of visceral fat increase we start depositing fat in the liver and muscle. We can see these effects even in some young people, using new medical imaging techniques. The fat deposited changes the way in which these organs work to regulate our metabolism. Again, one significant thing they do is interfere with the ability of insulin to work properly. When blood levels of cholesterol and fat are high, we even start to incorporate these molecules into the walls of our blood vessels and this leads to plaque formation—plaques are like scales on the inside of our blood vessels that interfere with their ordinary functioning and can form a focus for blood clots which can block the vessels. Blood vessels elsewhere can be affected; for example, fat-associated poor vascular function is an important reason for erectile failure in older men. The widely used drugs Viagra and Cialis work by opening the blood vessels up and sending blood to the penis, so it becomes more erect. Might this fact be marketed as an incentive for men to stay thin?

Because the wrong kind of fat in our cell membranes leads them to be stiffer, some hormones cannot do their jobs properly. Insulin made by the pancreas increases in the blood when blood glucose levels rise, because it stimulates the entry of glucose into cells—particularly in the muscle and liver where it is used by mitochondria as a fuel source. Our bodies are designed to use glucose as the primary source of fuel, with fat as the backup—just as hybrid cars are designed to use the battery first and fuel as the backup. But if our cells are not sensitive to insulin, we cannot use glucose as a fuel and its levels in the blood rise. When they remain high for too long the glucose joins to proteins in all sorts of tissues including blood vessels, nerves, and the kidneys, impairing their functions. This is why the complications of diabetes include blood vessel disease, heart attacks and strokes, nerve problems, and kidney failure. The eye is particularly sensitive to high levels of glucose affecting its blood vessels, nerve cells, and the lens. This risk of blindness is high in poorly controlled diabetes. Indeed the longer we have diabetes the more likely these complications become. Treating diabetes well is not easy—it involves drugs which are variably effective or, if the disease is severe enough, insulin injections. Diabetes of this type can be very problematic for both patient and doctor.

As for insulin, when cell membranes become affected by the wrong fats, leptin does not work well either. Because leptin naturally suppresses appetite, this dysfunction might exacerbate the problems associated with a high-fat diet by reducing satiety. Furthermore there are complex feedback links between insulin and leptin secretion. Once these systems become disturbed by impaired responses to these hormones, the risk of disease rises.

But fat tissue is more than just fat cells. Visceral fat contains immune cells that make inflammation-causing substances. So someone who has more visceral fat is likely to have a greater inflammatory profile. Inflammation is the process by which cells similar to the white cells of blood invade tissues and secrete chemicals and hormones which can damage neighbouring tissue. Inflammation is good when it surrounds a wound and kills invading bacteria to prevent infection, but it is not good when it attacks otherwise healthy tissue—for example our blood vessels or kidneys. The role of inflammation relative to the other mechanisms we have described in diabetes and cardiovascular disease is uncertain—but both are more likely if we have the wrong kind of obesity.

Obesity also leads to an increased risk of some cancers. It is not entirely clear why. Some hormones like oestrogen and progesterone are more soluble in fat than they are in water and so are found in greater concentrations in fat tissues. Hence fat can act as a store for these hormones and they can be metabolized inside fat into more active forms. This may explain why sex-hormone-sensitive cancers like post-menopausal breast cancer and uterine cancer are more common in obese women, although prostate cancer is not more common in obese men. But other cancers that are not obviously hormone sensitive are also more common in obese people, including kidney and colon cancer. Perhaps the answer to these differences in risk lies in changes in cellular response to growth hormones too—we need much more research here.

What we have described are ways in which obesity appears to lead directly to an increase in disease risk. But there are more indirect considerations we must not ignore. Obesity can be an indicator of other forms of unhealthy lifestyle and it may be that much of the disease risk associated with it results from these lifestyle factors.

Obesity may indicate an unhealthy diet, for example one high in so-called 'trans-fats'. These are an unusual form of unsaturated fat which is not healthy because it changes the concentrations of fat-protein complexes, leading to higher levels of the unhealthy form of cholesterol (LDL) versus the healthy form (HDL). There are small amounts of trans-fats in some milk, and in red meat, but the majority of trans-fats in our diets come from chemically processed foods in which the fat has been changed to make it stable.

But it goes beyond that. Research shows that people who have poor diets are also more likely to smoke and less likely to seek early medical advice if they become ill and it is sometimes difficult to determine which of these factors are most important, whether we are assessing cause or effect.

The 'metabolic syndrome' is the name given to the association between visceral obesity, unbalanced levels of fats in the bloodstream, and diabetes and cardiovascular disease. Not all elements need be present for someone to have the syndrome and indeed the relationship between them varies between individuals, both within and across populations. It is called a syndrome rather than a single disease because it is this collection of components which leads to the pathological condition and health risk to an individual. Sometimes the use of a word like 'syndrome' seems to be only a way of concealing our ignorance about what is really going on in a disease process. But while doctors and scientists argue about this in relation to the metabolic syndrome, it is becoming clear that in this case it is a set of health problems that often do go together. However, there may be one set of risk factors which leads to the syndrome in a particular person, and quite a different set in another person. This may make the problem hard to tackle, especially in terms of prevention, because the necessary measures will not be the same for everyone. This means that we have to look harder at the origins of the syndrome, and indeed of obesity itself. We will do this in the next chapter.

3

The Origins of Obesity

Nice and fat

There is more than one perspective on body shape. Throughout much of human history, body fat has been recognized as a sign of health and also as an indicator of social position. Venus figurines found in archaeological sites across Europe, and dating from between 20,000 and 35,000 years ago, depict very rotund female figures, and it is believed that these were probably Palaeolithic fertility symbols.

The singer and actress Jessica Simpson focused on some contemporary issues concerning fat in her documentary series *The Price of Beauty*. Is it a sign of beauty for a woman to be fat and, if so, how fat? In some parts of Africa young women are fed on high-fat foods until they become grossly obese, as this is thought to show that they are healthy and ready for marriage. Young women in rural Mauritania are sent to 'fattening farms' where they are beaten if they do not consume extraordinary amounts of fat-dense food. It is estimated that up to 20 per cent of young girls in rural Mauritania are subjected to this practice, known as *leblouh*. A typical diet for a six-year-old girl will include two cups of butter and 20 litres of camel's milk—every day. Some girls choke to death from being force-fed.

Similar practices occur in Uganda where young women are fattened up for two months prior to marriage—they are made to drink a jug of camel's milk every two hours and can put on up to 80 pounds. The presence of stretch marks on the abdomen is regarded as an essential beauty sign. Less extreme but similar practices are known in other parts of Africa. The strange thing is that while some body fat is essential for reproduction, gross obesity is associated with infertility.

These seem awful examples to people from developed countries. But in many highly developed societies, from the time of the Buddha in about 400 BC to contemporary life in cities in Asia, to be fat is seen as a sign of accomplishment, affluence, and social status. But then again, Western society has at times gone to extremes the other way. Why is it that the contemporary fashion industry promotes emaciated, gaunt, seemingly under-nourished skeletal figures as symbols of elegance and beauty? Not only is this an unrealistic physique in health terms, but thousands of girls have been harmed by the pressure to emulate this body image, which has led to eating disorders such as anorexia and bulimia and also—again—to infertility. None of these examples seems to make much biological sense.

Humans are designed to have some body fat. Even the fittest of individuals needs some fat to provide the energy reserves necessary for coping with normal life. But while good nutrition is clearly a sign of health and thus fertility, we now live in a very different world where excess body fat is associated with disease. At the centre of the crisis is the dramatic change in the number of people suffering from diabetes and cardiovascular disease. In this chapter we will explain why this has happened.

The amounts of fat in our bodies change throughout our lives. We described the striking observation that the fattest babies in the animal kingdom are human babies. We suggested that this gives the baby a fuel store, which is needed because the human brain grows most rapidly in the first two years after birth. Infants gradually get thinner up to the age of about three, then they start putting on body fat again until about six years of age (at least in modern societies). We will come back to the importance of this childhood weight gain later.

Nearly all of us tend to put on a little weight in middle age, partly because we exercise less, and partly because the ageing process affects some of our control systems, especially the accuracy of the body's fat controller. But in between these two time points—the other five ages of man in Shakespeare's terms—we should remain reasonably thin and with a stable level of body fat. But observation of contemporary societies reveals something else: most of us just go on getting fatter as we get older.

Weight for height

How do we measure fatness? There are several ways. The most sophisticated use X-ray or magnetic resonance scanners to calculate the amount of fat, muscle, and bone as a per centage of total body weight. A typical healthy male might be about 13–17 per cent fat and a typical healthy female 20–21 per cent, because women have some additional fat deposited on their hips and in their breasts. But such techniques are restricted largely to medical research; most estimates of fatness (also called adiposity) are made simply by measuring height and weight.

The most widely used measure for adults is the body mass index (BMI). This is calculated as the weight of the individual (in kilograms) divided by their height (in metres) squared. For Western adults a BMI less than 18.5 kg/m^2 is regarded as too thin; a normal BMI is between 18.5 and 24.9 kg/m^2. The term 'overweight' is restricted technically to those having a BMI between 25 and 30 and the term 'obese' to those with a BMI over 30 kg/m^2. But these categories differ between populations. In Asian populations, a higher disease risk can be seen even at BMIs as low as 22 kg/m².

The BMI and these definitions are those used in international comparisons so we will use them in this book. The BMI, however, has serious limitations. As it relies only on height and weight it cannot separate out the amount of fat, muscle, and bone. A very fit rugby player, perhaps a first row prop forward, may have lots of muscle and little fat. But because he weighs more than average his BMI may be close to 30 even though he is in fact perfectly healthy.

Before 1980, the percentage of people who were overweight was much lower, although even then we knew that it was increasing. But now the problem has spiralled massively upwards, so that the proportion of overweight and obese people in Asian populations has more than doubled: 50 per cent or more of the population can now be classified as overweight. The problem is even more acute in developing countries. In Brazil the obesity rate nearly doubled in women and tripled in men between 1975 and 2003. Similar effects have been observed in India, with a doubling over ten years, and in China, where it has tripled even though the absolute rate still remains low. In developing countries the rise in obesity is faster than in the West and is particularly striking in urban areas.

The World Health Organization projects that by 2015, 2.3 billion adults worldwide will be overweight and more than 700 million will be obese. Almost a third of teenagers are now overweight in the United States and one-quarter are clinically obese. The effect is occurring earlier and earlier in our lives too. Now the fat of middle age is spilling over into childhood, adolescence, and young adult life.

The statistics for non-communicable diseases associated with obesity are even more worrying. They account for 36 million deaths per year, nearly two-thirds of all deaths globally, from whatever cause. In China it is estimated that there are over 100 million diabetics.

And diabetes and cardiovascular disease are setting in earlier and earlier in our lives. In urban parts of India, as many as 20 per cent of 30-year-olds have diabetes.

Evolution never prepared us for this

So why do so many people now get fat and suffer the direct and indirect consequences of obesity? The simple answer is that the way we live our lives has changed dramatically in at least three ways—what we eat, what we do, and how we live our lives. We need to dissect out each of these differences. In doing so we will expose the problems of some widely held assumptions and some rather naive thinking.

Our starting point is human evolution. In our book *Mismatch* we explained that our biology has been shaped over more than 100,000 years by selection and other evolutionary processes. These matched our biology to our world, but of course this was a very different world from the one we now inhabit. It is in the nature of evolutionary processes that they set the range of biological responses that we can make to an environmental change. But that range has limits. We cannot cope with an environmental change which is too large or beyond our ancestral experience. If our ancestors did not experience certain environmental conditions, they could not have undergone selection to leave us with a biology which allows us to cope with them now.

A good example concerns the level of oxygen in the air. All our early ancestors lived at altitudes below about 3,500 m. So it is not surprising that in general human beings can cope with altitudes up to that level. It takes some of us a few days before we are comfortable if we go from sea level to a mountain resort at 3,500 m, but most of us can do it. However, no human society can survive successfully above about 4,000 m. Very fit individuals may be able to climb higher than this, even without oxygen—for example, to work in mines at 4,500 m in the Andes for a short period of time—but even then, these individuals

44

will have to descend to lower altitudes before too long. Human fertility also falls off dramatically with altitude, so we clearly never evolved to colonize these lofty regions of the planet. One way of putting this is to say that we are just not 'designed' to live at these high altitudes—but evolution has no design or purpose, and does not imply that a designer exists. But contrast humans with the bar-headed goose which can fly at 10,000 m—needless to say without oxygen tanks. So some species have evolved to be adapted to life at great heights and low oxygen levels, but we are not one of them.

We find it very useful to take this evolutionary perspective in order to understand why the changes in what we eat, what we do, and how we live our lives have had such dramatic consequences. Diet and lifestyle are important aspects of the environment which we have made and now inhabit.

The most common explanation for the rise in obesity is that we have adopted a lifestyle in which we eat far too much of the wrong kinds of food and are too lazy to take physical exercise—we are guilty of the sins of gluttony and sloth. Some public health experts try to make us feel guilty about this. There is of course a degree of truth in their charge because it is not possible to become obese without taking on board more energy from the food we eat than we expend through basal metabolism, growth, physical activity, and even reproduction.

But there is much more to the story than that. We need to unpack it, to see what is involved. First, it is true that modern diets, especially in the developed world, often contain high levels of sugars or carbohydrates which are highly refined—such as in white bread, sweet drinks, and polished rice—and these foods release their carbohydrates into the bloodstream very rapidly. They push up blood glucose levels quickly, and are consequently called 'high glycaemic index' foods. The high levels of glucose in the bloodstream are more than the body can easily use as an immediate fuel source, so they push up the blood levels of insulin; the excess fuel is taken up by adipose and other tissues to be stored as fat. This is a simple and highly effective strategy, which evolved in most animals including even some insects, whereby fat storage provides a depot of energy which can be used later.

Got too much on your plate? Well, gobble it up anyway and stash some away for later; you never know when your next meal is going to come along. This biology is widespread. Laboratory animals fed on high-glycaemic-index foods get fat. So do cats, dogs, and other pets, such as budgerigars and gerbils. Animals do not get fat in the wild, however, except those which lay down extra fat before going into hibernation. So there must be something unnatural about the fat family dog. It is strange that so many scientists still stick to the view that because obesity runs in families, inherited genetic effects must hold the key—but how do they explain that often the dog in these families is obese too?

There are other unfortunate things about modern Western diets. For example they contain relatively low levels of fibre, especially if they have a high refined carbohydrate content. Fibre is useful because it retains nutrients in the gut and so delays their absorption. Hence a given caloric load in a meal that contains high fibre produces a lower level of blood glucose over a longer period of time than one which does not.

Then of course there is the fat content of the food we consume. Many modern foods contain high levels of saturated fats in meat, eggs, and dairy produce. Snacks such as biscuits, chocolates, cakes, and crisps often have a high fat content too. Unfortunately, because we eat them between meals, they tend to alter the body's metabolism in favour of fat deposition. And modern processed food sometimes contains different fats, such as trans-fats, which in the past we only ate in tiny quantities because we had not invented the industrial processes for producing them.

Modern Western diets are unbalanced in other respects too. Even the trace nutrients that we need in our diet, such as iron and zinc, folic acid and vitamins, are sometimes not present in high enough concentrations to keep us healthy. Vegetarians can be deficient in vitamin B12, which is found primarily in meat—this is a major problem in some ethnic groups in India which have very strict vegetarian diets.

We are a generalist species, in other words one which can survive on a wide range of diets. Otherwise we would not have been able to inhabit the globe in the way that we do, from the Tropics to the Arctic regions. The Inuit eat large quantities of meat, yet many people in India are strict vegetarians. But this does not take away from the fact that it is the balance of nutrients as well as their absolute amounts in our diet which is so important to our health.

And so, now that we can see how the components of the modern diet fit into the story, we return to our evolutionary perspective.

While there is still room for some speculation and it is dangerous to generalize because our ancestors lived in so many different ways, there is a general consensus about the kinds of diet our predecessors had. The diets of hunter-gatherers in our Palaeolithic past 100,000 years ago contained very few simple carbohydrates, let alone sugars other than perhaps from wild honey and the fructose in fruits. The meat content in their diets may have been high but it was usually lean meat, because the animals that were hunted for food ran around even more than their early human predators. The balance of the diet was made up of a higher proportion of vegetables, roots, nuts, and seeds than most people consume today, even in developing countries.

And so we evolved largely with a metabolism designed around a kind of high-fibre, low-glycaemic-index diet. There were times of year when there was perhaps more access to fat in the game hunted—which provided a welcome high-energy storage form of fuel. When that happened the hunter-gatherers would gorge themselves to store up excess fuel for harder times. Even in more recent historical times, the Plains Indians of North America were known to engage in this kind of gorging behaviour after mass buffalo kills at a time of the year when the animals were well-fed and relatively fat. It seems that we, like other species, evolved to be able to store fat when food supplies are in excess so that we can cope better in hard times.

Modern times

Over the last 10,000 years our lives have changed considerably, but our biology has changed much less. Evolutionary change is generally a slow process. Starting about 10,000 years ago in the Middle East, we invented agriculture and learnt how to herd goats, sheep, and cattle. These skills also developed independently in other parts of the world. Agriculture and animal husbandry gradually changed what we ate. For example, with the domestication of cattle in some parts of the world, we started to drink cow's milk. In those places we developed the enzymes needed to break down milk sugar (lactose) in the gut. However, in Asia, the Americas, and large parts of Africa, where cows were not farmed for milk, a tolerance of lactose never evolved. Many people from these regions still cannot consume cow's milk without becoming sick.

But while the development of agriculture produced a big change, it was small compared to the changes in our diets over the past 200 years. The industrial revolution brought with it an agricultural revolution, which gave us a greater dependence on large-scale farming of grain, corn, sugar cane, and beet. The industrial revolution also saw the dawn of the modern food-processing industry. Food changed from being composed of simple natural ingredients to increasingly processed and refined products. Salt, sugar, and fats were added to improve taste and preserve the food. The food industry grew as cities expanded, so that fewer and fewer people across the planet could grow their own food. The relationship between food as it was sold and its original ingredients became more remote. In the 1860s,

Emperor Louis Napoleon III of France offered a prize for the development of a substitute for butter suitable for use by the armed forces and the lower social classes (don't ask what went into the winning recipe), and since then synthetic spreads and cooking oils have become a common part of our diet. For many years some processed foods have contained trans-fats, which were a direct result of the processing of the ingredients. Corn oil and corn starch became nearly universal ingredients, and so fructose and omega-6 fatty acid levels in foods started to rise.

Then along came the fast food industry, the soft drink industry, our expanded intake of confectionary and alcohol—all excess calories that are easier to turn into fat than energy. And the cheapest foods now are often those that are most calorie-dense—so the more impoverished people in our societies eat less balanced diets than those who are better off.

Technology has changed our lives in other ways too, of course. Few of us now hunt or fish to feed ourselves or wander the forests in search of tubers and seeds. Fewer and fewer of us even walk to a shop to buy our food—we are more likely to drive or to take a bus or train, or just to pick up the phone or order online. Manual work is increasingly replaced by machines. Leisure is spent in front of a computer or television, rather than walking or playing a game or a sport outside. Our children are more likely to be driven to school than to walk or ride a bike.

Of course we do not know how much energy our hunter-gatherer ancestors expended each day—some anthropologists think that it was much more than we do now; others are less certain. The estimates are based on hunter-gatherer communities which still exist, but they have changed their lifestyles over the last 10,000 years too, and many of them are not free of modern influences. But if we look at more recent times, the situation is clearer. Most of us expend much less energy in living our lives than our great-grandparents did a century ago. Studies in countries such as Japan show a direct correlation between the number of motor cars and the number of people who are obese. Other studies find the same correlations with the average number of hours spent watching television. While it is tempting to draw a cause and effect relationship, there is considerable debate about this. Would increasing exercise at a population level reduce the rate of obesity? Logic suggests that it would, although the size of the effect may be much smaller than might be expected—for reasons which will become apparent.

We have grown up eating three meals every day with one or two snacks in between them. It was somewhat different in Victorian times, as many people had large meals at breakfast and in the evening but little for lunch. But as we now live and work in heated buildings and need to metabolize very little to keep warm, and as many of us spend our working days and leisure time sitting and being transported about the world by mechanical means, we can see how easily a mismatch between what we eat and how we burn it up can occur.

Active kids

Many parents bemoan the fact that children just do not seem to engage in as much physical activity at school as they did when they were children themselves. It is true that in the UK, for example, many local education authorities have sold off fields where children could engage in sport or just run around. Very often they are valuable pieces of real estate and the cash helps to balance the books of the local council. In addition, the number of children who walk or cycle to school is far lower than it used to be. Parents worry about traffic or potential molestation by paedophiles or just that, if their children are making their own way home from school, it is hard to know exactly what they might get up to on the way. There is no doubting the seriousness of the road traffic accident worry and very few Western cities have adequate cycle lanes or paths which would allow children to go to and from school in relative safety. The statistics, however, do not bear out the worry about other threats—it seems that children are no more likely to be murdered, abducted, or sexually assaulted today than they were a generation ago.

But of course children don't need acres of space in order to exercise. What about good old-fashioned physical education lessons? These still take place in many schools and are prescribed in most curricula. They were never the most popular lessons among many children. Now they are deeply unfashionable with some groups, who effectively refuse to participate. The difference in perception occurs in the early puberty years when boys and girls tend to separate in their attitudes. If there is a training element which seems linked to sporting or other prowess, the activity can often be sold to the boys in the class, but for the girls the concept of changing into unappealing or revealing sports kit and then getting hot and sweaty is not alluring.

But what about life outside school? Recent studies suggest that this too may be important, although the reliability of such studies is uncertain. There are often very big differences between what people say they do and what they actually do, as measured by using electronic monitoring equipment. Nevertheless it is sobering to note that some researchers found that children who undertook a high level of physical activity at school were far less likely to be physically active at home. In contrast, those children who appeared to do relatively little physical exercise at school were more likely to go out to play football or join dance classes outside school hours. So in the end the net effect may be the same for both groups.

This is not to say that children do not differ in the overall amounts of physical activity in which they engage over the course of a week and that possibly this may link to how well they control their appetites and body weight. But what these studies do suggest is that the setting for physical activity is established relatively early in the lives of our children. If we force them to do more exercise in one setting—say at school—will they do less in another? Once again we get the feeling that merely focusing on exercise levels in children is not the whole answer. Exercise may help but it may also be too late to produce a permanent change, at least in some people. One of our major themes pops up again—people vary.

The energy that we expend in deliberate physical activity is only part of the story. Jogging or weightlifting is all very well and certainly burns up calories, but recent research suggests a surprising way in which we also use calories. Ever noticed that the nervous, twitchy child in the class, who is always fidgeting and shifting in his or her seat, dropping things on the floor and picking them up, is also likely to be the thin child? They are not going anywhere or doing anything very useful but they are burning up a lot of energy in the process. This type of apparently minor activity uses a lot of energy every day, but once again it balances out. If we exercise in the gym on the way home from work, we will probably fidget less later when we are sitting in front of the computer.

Once again our biology seems designed to defeat weight loss. But of course this is the wrong way of looking at it. Our biology has evolved to do just that—to keep our body weight fairly constant regardless of what our level of activity actually is by adjusting a range of processes which consume energy. Indeed there are aspects of our biology designed to favour laying down energy reserves. This is because in our evolutionary past obesity was rare and there was always an advantage in storing those excess calories for a rainy day. We are left with this fundamental property of our biology. Metabolic processes which were useful 10,000 years ago are one reason why we are in trouble now.

Short lives

How long do we think our Palaeolithic ancestors lived? We don't know precisely, but fossil records give us some clues. On average their lifespan might have been as little as 30 years from birth, but this figure is heavily influenced by the high rate of infant mortality. Probably only about half the babies born survived, most dying soon after birth or at weaning, with others perishing in childhood. It may be that, provided they lived beyond childhood, there was a reasonable chance of their living to a much older age. Once again, however, it is clear that average life expectancy has changed dramatically in more recent times. In France in 1800 a man had a life expectancy at birth of about 30; in 1900 this was 45, in 1950 about 64, and now he can expect to live until about 78 (longer for a woman). The same trends, albeit with different baselines, have been observed in the USA, the UK, and many other developed countries. And many developing countries have seen major changes in life expectancy too—for example, in India there was on average a 13 per cent increase in life expectancy in men in the last 25 years of the 20th century.

If we now live longer lives than we did in our evolutionary past, then health problems which evolution was never able to filter out will emerge in later life. Indeed this is one of the most fundamental principles of evolutionary biology—selection pressures are strongest in the period up to when reproductive capacity is maximal. This is because in the end evolution is driven by successful reproduction. Ageing is a process whereby repair mechanisms, needed to protect the individual up to the age of reproduction, are overwhelmed by the accumulated damage from toxins, solar and cosmic radiation, and other factors. Once reproduction is over, the evolutionary pressures to repair cells are greatly reduced. So we can expect that as we age, the pressures of metabolic overload induced by changed diets and exercise patterns are more likely to be exposed in the form of obesity and chronic disease—for example diabetes and vascular damage, which lead to heart disease and stroke. The risk of mutation increases, and as DNA repair processes wane, cancer becomes more likely.

From the evolutionary point of view extreme fatness would have been rare, but in contrast a moderate level of body fat is good for survival, for reproduction, and even for defence against infection. But because our Palaeolithic ancestors lived shorter lives, the diabetes of today's middle-aged obese person was not a problem they faced. So at its simplest it is the concatenation of longer lives and different lifestyles today, mismatched to our evolved fundamental biology, which is associated with the current increased level of diabetes and cardiovascular disease.

The consequence of this argument is that, if only we could restore our diets and behaviour to those for which our evolution suits us, we would stay slim and be incredibly healthy. Reducing the glycaemic index of foods is partly the basis of the Atkins diet (there is another component of it relating to appetite control which we will return to later) and there are many other dietary fads and supplements which purport to be as effective. Some of them are indeed effective, at least in the short term—but there is the rub. For some reason people who restrict themselves to such diets lose weight for a period of time, but then they inevitably pile back on the pounds. It is as if an individual's metabolism has been set to achieve a certain body weight, and while it will allow the body to deviate from this over a short period of time if the person decides to consume a different diet, it will not allow the body weight to fall by too much for too long even though being overweight may be associated in the long term with poor health.

As we progress through this book we will add other layers of complexity to the story. If we do not view the full picture in proper perspective we will never find the right solutions. We started from the immediate problem—something very much in the foreground of the picture—that although we have to eat too much and exercise too little to become obese, dieting and exercise do not restore healthy body weight in everybody. People are different. Two people may live in exactly the same way but one becomes fat and the other does not; one gets diabetes while the other continues to control their blood glucose very well. In this chapter we have added the evolutionary perspective to our picture. It helps us to get a clearer idea of how our fundamental biological processes contribute to the problems we now face. But still the picture is far from complete. We will have to keep filling it in if we are to come up with some effective solutions.

4

Now We Are Sick

What is normal?

The diseases we are concerned with in this book, particularly diabetes and cardiovascular disease, often creep up on us. We are concerned with the emergence of type 2 diabetes, which is generally much more insidious, unlike that of insulin-dependent (type 1) diabetes, which usually starts with an acute episode—sometimes even loss of consciousness. Many people have it without knowing, and it is only when they have their blood sugar levels checked that they find that they suffer from this disease. Similarly, while some people discover they have cardiovascular disease when they have a heart attack or a stroke, a thorough medical examination would usually have uncovered high blood pressure or altered blood lipid levels well before these more serious events occurred. A very high proportion of people have such signs but know nothing about it. One of the problems of this subtle appearance of disease is how to define when disease is present.

Not only can individuals be unaware of these health problems but so too can public health organizations. Just recently, in 2010, the estimate of the number of people with diabetes in China had to be revised upward dramatically. As more information became available it was found that the previous estimate of 45 million was far too low. Indeed official figures suggest that there are now about 100 million people in China with diabetes and this may still be an underestimate. Getting accurate figures is impossible unless extensive population studies are undertaken.

Thousands of pages in medical journals have been filled with debate and discussion about how best to define diseases such as diabetes or hypertension. The problem is that there is not a sharp dividing line between normal and abnormal—and what is healthy for one individual may be unhealthy for another. It is easy to say whether or not a person has a broken leg, or whether or not your child has measles. It is much more difficult when ill health which may have had its roots in childhood (or even before) emerges over many years.

The question is made more complex because what may start as very subtle changes such as thickening of the walls of our blood vessels, which we know can even be present in quite young children, does not emerge as high blood pressure or heart disease until decades later. And how rapidly these clinical conditions emerge may be influenced by many things, such as how much we exercise, what we eat, how stressful our jobs or our personal lives are, and, as we shall see in later chapters, by other biological factors such as our genetic and epigenetic make-up.

So when does a person move from being healthy to being unhealthy? We could say that they are unhealthy as soon as their physiology indicates a deviation from normal, even if they do not show any signs of disease. On the other hand we could wait until the person's productivity and quality of life are affected—perhaps following a heart attack or angina or a stroke—but isn't that shutting the stable door after the horse has bolted? So the answer must lie somewhere in between, when some threshold of abnormality is reached—say in blood levels of the markers of inflammatory processes which are part of the disease process. In practice this is the sort of definition that is generally used—but only after a lengthy academic discourse allows a consensus to be reached on what is normal and what is not in terms of the choice of such markers and their levels.

While we need to have some working definitions, there is a flawed set of concepts underlying the problem. We are dealing with a broad and continuous range of possible measurements. Consider adult height in men—obviously it varies considerably. Furthermore the average height of a man from Holland is different from the average height of an Inuit man from Northern Canada. One is tall and thin, the other short and stocky. Not only is the average height different but so is the range of heights observed. We can imagine that there will be more extremely tall men in Holland than on Baffin Island, and that in absolute centimetres we would find a greater percentage of men under the height of 160 cm on Baffin Island than in Amsterdam. And if we compared them with men from the Efe, a pygmy tribe from the Congo, a short Inuit man might be considered a tall by the Efe man.

So what constitutes an abnormally short male? We can see that no definition based simply on height makes sense. It clearly depends on ancestral background—whether a man is an Inuit, a Dutchman, or an Efe. It also depends on his parents—short parents tend to have short children and tall parents tall children, because genetic influences are involved. So we might expect that if a very short Dutch man married a very short Dutch woman, their offspring will be at the short end of the height range. So does this make the short Dutch man abnormal? Statistically he may be right at the lower end of the range of heights seen in Holland: 99 per cent of the male population may be taller, but this still does not make him 'abnormal'. After all, somebody has to be at the extreme end of the normal range—just as someone has to be the oldest person in the world on any one day. But it is also possible that he does have a biological problem which is affecting his growth. There are genetically transmitted forms of short stature—achondroplasia is one example—so perhaps the Dutch man's family has heritable achondroplasia. Achondroplastics are easy to recognize—they are very short people with relatively large trunks and heads and very short arms and legs. But there are also much more subtle genetic defects that lead to short stature without obvious skeletal abnormality.

So when we talk about the 'normal range' for height, it is a purely statistical definition taken from measuring lots of people—it says nothing about whether people outside this range are abnormal. To determine this we have to do more tests or examine them in some other way.

Equally, a person may have a height well within the normal range but still be abnormal. The individual may be a respectable 175 cm tall but have had very tall parents. When we examine him or her carefully we may find that he or she has coeliac disease which impairs digestion. The individual has had his or her growth affected and has not grown to full genetic potential. Yet from a purely statistical measure of height he or she appears normal.

The point we are making is that whenever we have a continuous measure—that is one which does not break down into discrete compartments like fractured or intact, male or female—then definitions become statistical. We can be fairly certain whether or not an individual has a broken leg without needing to compare him or her to others. But just knowing someone's height tells us little about their normality or health without a lot more information. It gets very complex when we start looking at the pathways to diabetes and cardiovascular disease.

We believe that it is not the presence or absence of an abnormal finding that defines the risk of diabetes and cardiovascular disease; rather it is the pattern of the life-course of the individual, and his or her particular context, that puts him or her at greater risk. This is a new concept, and one of great importance, but it also sits uneasily with doctors who are more used to traditional diagnostic approaches. A patient complains of pain in the chest. Is it indigestion—yes or no? Is it a heart attack—yes or no?

Living longer in the developed world

Diabetes and cardiovascular disease have long been recognized as problems of the developed world. For many years they were seen to be diseases of affluence because they appeared to be predominant in richer countries. But within these countries it is actually the poorer, more disadvantaged people who are now more at risk. There are many reasons why this is the case—cheaper foods tend to be less healthy, socio-economically disadvantaged people face barriers in accessing healthcare rapidly, and they are more likely to smoke.

They are also more likely to have jobs in which their autonomy is limited. Recent studies by Sir Michael Marmot of public servants in the UK and population groups in eastern Europe show that ill health is more likely in people with less control over their lives. So people who worked in jobs where they simply had to do what they were told, with little opportunity to show initiative or flexibility, were more likely to have heart disease and other chronic illnesses. In Marmot's study lower-ranking civil servants in the UK were more at risk than higher-ranking colleagues. As we shall see in later chapters, this does not just apply to the UK, because poorer, less educated people in many countries live in cycles of disadvantage which affect their health in successive generations.

In a typical Western country about half of us can expect to die of cardiovascular disease. But we will do so at an advanced age, unless we are unlucky or poor, because our healthcare services can provide drugs, surgery, stents to keep blocked arteries open, and even heart transplants. Of course this effort consumes large sums of money—between

5 and 15 per cent of an advanced country's GDP goes into providing health services late in an individual's life. Our societies value this investment as a social good because we now live much healthier, productive, and enjoyable lives well into our post-retirement years. It is also an economic good because over the past two decades improvements in healthcare and public health measures such as reducing smoking have delayed the appearance of cardiovascular disease until much later in life. This in turn has led many Western governments to consider raising the statutory age of retirement—which is helpful for them in tough economic times.

But there is a growing concern that, with the rising epidemic of abdominal obesity, the gains may be reversed. Could it be that we will again start seeing heart disease at an earlier age? There are respected researchers who argue that this is indeed the case. If they are right we may see life expectancy, which has risen progressively across developed nations, start to decline again. Children born today may not live as long as their parents.

One frightening hint comes from studies of diabetes in Western countries. Type 2 diabetes used to be called 'maturity onset diabetes' because 40 years ago it generally appeared in the sixth or seventh decade of life. Seeing an adolescent who had type 2 diabetes was very rare. But now in a typical paediatric diabetic clinic almost half of new patients will have type 2 diabetes—the term 'maturity onset' is no longer meaningful.

The longer a person has type 2 diabetes, the more likely the nasty complications of heart problems, blindness, and kidney disease are to occur. Even with good diabetic control—and that is not as easy as it sounds—complications will appear if the person lives long enough. So if the disease starts four decades earlier than it used to, we can anticipate more complications in the later, but still potentially productive, years of our lives. We are worried by this trend, and so are paediatricians and doctors throughout the Western world.

A new kind of transition in the developing world

We are used to thinking of the diseases of the developing world as being associated with under-nutrition and infection. And sadly, it is true that almost a billion people around the world still struggle to have sufficient food and adequate nutrition. Too many children in Africa, Asia, and Latin America grow up stunted, a sign of chronic under-nutrition and ill health. Malaria, tuberculosis, polio, bilharzia, and many other tropical infections still affect millions of people, with potentially horrific consequences. Even the most basic aspects of public health and medical care are absent for many people. Clean water is unheard of in some places. Nearly half a million women die each year in pregnancy or childbirth, reflecting the lack of the most basic obstetric and midwifery services, and each year some 8 million children die before their fifth birthday—largely in Africa and southern Asia.

This is the classic picture we all have of the pattern of disease in developing countries. But that picture is incomplete. For in the last two decades we have seen the start of a new epidemic in these countries: of diabetes and cardiovascular disease and other complications of obesity. Indeed it is now estimated that almost as many people in the developing world suffer from these chronic diseases—which many of us think of as resulting from excess—as from under-nutrition. And cancer, allergic disease, and senile dementia are also rising rapidly in developing countries. Up to 20 times as many people globally die from non-communicable disease as from HIV. But what is frightening is that the rate of diabetes and cardiovascular disease is rising rapidly. The predictions of future incidence, while astronomical, are in our view likely to be underestimates.

Some hospitals in Beijing report rates of diabetes in pregnancy of more than 20 per cent. Indeed across Asia the rate of diabetes in pregnancy has risen dramatically. As diabetes in pregnancy is an early warning of diabetes exploding in a population, we think that, unchecked, the rate of diabetes in China will rise dramatically in the next two decades from its already alarming level. The same is true of India. Even in Africa, the continent of under-nutrition, rates of diabetes and heart disease are rising, particularly in populations migrating from the countryside to cities such as Lagos. Some of the highest rates of diabetes are on small island states such as Nauru, where more than 40 per cent of the adult population can be affected.

As in developed countries, diabetes and cardiovascular heart disease are appearing in people in developing countries at relatively young ages. For example, in India more than 60 per cent of newly diagnosed diabetics are under the age of 50, and 25 per cent are in their thirties. Such an early onset will impact on the quality of life of entire families as well as putting impossible burdens on rudimentary health systems and impeding economic development. The implications of all of this for trying to close the so-called North–South divide—a symbol of the health inequalities across the globe—are extremely worrying. This is why the British Commonwealth nations at their 2009 meeting of heads of state in Trinidad and Tobago urged action to be taken. In response to this, Ban Ki-moon, the United Nations Secretary General, called a special General Assembly Summit in 2011 to address the issues of non-communicable disease in the developing world. And that is one of the reasons we have written this book.

One driver of this epidemic is obvious. The nature of the food consumed has changed. From eating unrefined foods, many people across the developing world are now turning to high-fat, refined foods for their basic diet. Foods are increasingly cooked in corn oil. And just as in the West, the cheapest foods are often the most energy-dense, with a high glycaemic index. The problem is aggravated by mass migrations from rural areas to cities. In rural settings, subsistence agriculture provides foods which are unlikely to exceed our metabolic capacity, especially as the rural lifestyle is often associated with high levels of physical activity. But in cities these simple staples are often replaced by sweet drinks and fried food. This is a one-way process. As countries move through the economic transition they also move through this nutritional transition. Indeed in countries such as China, India, and Indonesia the rate of the rise in diabetes and cardiovascular disease correlates well with the economic growth of the country.

What does it all cost? This may seem a cynical question. Health and disease are about far more than just dollars. They are often about lives lived happily or ruined. But governments and agencies have to work in dollars because what they can do is essentially limited by resource allocation. Non-communicable diseases account for about 35 million deaths a year globally—that is more than one every second of every minute of every hour of every day of the year.

In 2009 the World Economic Forum calculated that there is a real chance that the likely cost of non-communicable diseases could approach close to several trillion dollars a year. Furthermore, they concluded that both the likelihood and the severity of detrimental consequences of non-communicable diseases are increasing. The numbers are astronomical, whether we look at developed or developing countries, and the argument for doing something about them is obvious—the question is, what? This enormous burden of disease is not going away; in fact it is getting worse year on year, and especially in the parts of the world least able to deal with it.

The Millennium Development Goals

In 2000 the world's leaders adopted a grand vision for the least developed world. They agreed to a set of goals to be achieved by 2015. These Millennium Development Goals were designed to put pressure on developed countries to assist the developing world in making advances, and to indicate to governments and agencies some simple measurable priorities. These Millennium Development Goals include some fundamental targets such as eradicating extreme hunger and poverty (easy to say but hard to achieve), promoting maternal and child health, and providing universal primary education.

Progress on some of these goals has been slow and in 2010, when an audit was made, the failure to progress adequately on many of them was lamented. This has led to renewed commitments to address issues such as maternal and child health. For example, the 1,000 Days campaign launched by Hillary Clinton aims to improve child nutrition from conception through to two years of age, so as to promote a healthier start to life.

But it seems to us strange that, despite the scale of the problem which they represent, non-communicable diseases were not part of the Millennium Development Goals. Nowhere in the list of aims, which politicians, scientists, doctors, religious leaders, and educa tors drew up in the months leading up to January 2000, did non-communicable diseases make an appearance. It was almost as if the problem didn't exist.

Why?

Perhaps it was too hard. Addressing this issue is complex, and besides, it is not as politically appealing to some member states as dealing with maternal mortality in relation to childbirth or gender inequality. Achiev ing the Millennium Development Goals is a necessary condition for progress towards global equality but it is doubtful that this is realistically possible unless we also ensure that the adult population is healthy and productive. Economic progress is necessary for social progress.

Perhaps the challenge posed by non-communicable diseases arose too quickly for even the most flexible and manoeuvrable of medical research or healthcare organizations to cope with. This is not helped by the fact that we did not recognize that the disease epidemic was developing fastest in unexpected places, such as sub-Saharan Africa, one of the poorest regions on Earth. And lastly, we really had very little idea what to do about it. An inability to address a problem soon leads to a sense of resignation.

So what's new? We know that many readers will feel that they have heard all this before. Diabetes and cardiovascular disease are a problem whether you live in Manhattan or Bamako. We all know that if you eat a healthy diet and exercise more the problem will go away—won't it? There have been many books and endless articles and television programmes on the problem of obesity and its consequences. Officials from Departments of Health around the world have emphasized that this is a major problem which requires urgent attention. Politicians have thumped their lecterns in political speeches and vowed that something *will* be done about it. Parents and teachers have been encouraged to play their part in reversing the trend and helping tomorrow's children to be thinner and healthier. To be honest, we are all getting rather tired of hearing about this and just wish that the problem would go away. So why hasn't it?

5

The Thin Line

Slimming down

Many of us have tried to lose weight, and have failed to keep the lost kilograms off. This is probably why there are an extraordinary number of 'experts' who claim to be able to help us. Amazon.com currently lists more than 22,000 different books about weight loss—many of them claiming their own special way of guaranteeing success. And along with all this advice from the gurus in their books and magazine articles there is an enormous industry of weight loss regimes, very often based on the purchase of expensive diets, treatment, or advice sessions—it's a huge industry. The plethora of different approaches suggests that there is both a real problem to be addressed and an enormous marketing opportunity.

Why is the weight loss industry so big? Partly because so many people are indeed overweight or obese—or at least would like to look different. But the underlying reason is that losing weight is hard and these so-called 'cures' usually don't work—or, if they do work, do so only for a short time, after which the unhappy slimmer gains weight and is soon back to where he or she started. All of this is of course great for the weight loss industry. 'You have tried three different diets and none of them worked? Ah, well, that is because the ones you tried were not right for you. Instead this is the one for you ... sorry it's a bit more expensive', and so on.

And commercially marketed diets and programmes are only part of the story—there is the question of exercise. There is an increasing number of pseudo-exercise devices that claim to help us lose weight by some less energetic means—'three minutes a day will be enough ...'—when the simple logic is obvious: exercise largely works by burning calories and by changing aspects of our metabolism by inducing more muscle to be built. And there is no way to burn calories except by putting in the effort. Jogging for half an hour a day for an average man probably only burns off up to 400 calories, and a kilogram of fat has almost 8,000 calories in it! There is simply no way a very short period of exercise can replace prolonged effort which burns off fat and builds up muscle and sets it to work. And it turns out that building up the muscle is an important part of the story—for this reduces the chances of insulin resistance and slows the pathway to diabetes and cardiovascular disease.

Nevertheless, despite all the disappointments and all the money wasted on the latest diet or gadget, the orthodox view persists that losing weight, and consequently reducing one's disease risk, is simply a question of mind over matter, of willpower. Eat less or differently, exercise more, and avoid smoking, and we will be all right. This is all we have to do—do it and we will beat the global problem of diabetes and cardiovascular disease and we will all look, and be, healthy. We still read somewhere every day, somewhat to our frustration, that beating obesity and therefore the risk of non-communicable disease is simply a matter of eating fewer calories than we expend—so eating less and more wisely and exercising more will solve the problem. And if it doesn't? Well then the answer is obvious—it is our own fault!

But now we know that the picture is not so black and white.

Going native

As we described in Chapter 3, it is likely that if we all ate and lived as our ancestors did 20,000 years ago very few of us would be obese, and chronic disease would be very rare. We even have modern examples of this. The Pima Indians are a tribe who live in Mexico and also in Arizona. Many of those Pima who live in Mexico have lifestyles involving hard physical work in growing their food. They eat subsistence diets. Their level of obesity, diabetes, and cardiovascular disease is relatively low, at least compared to their northern cousins. In contrast, the Pima of Arizona live on reservations with high incomes from casinos and other enterprises, and lead very sedentary lives. They eat very energy-dense, high-glycaemic North American diets, rich in fats and refined sugars. They have some of the highest rates of diabetes and heart disease and obesity known—so high that it was thought for a long time that they had a special genetic defect. But what we can see is that two genetically very similar groups of people, of the same tribal origin, have very different rates of diabetes and cardiovascular disease because they have two very different lifestyles.

But while this sounds simple, a central feature of the human condition is that our culture and society also continue to evolve. We are not living in the Neolithic Stone Age and it is unrealistic to imagine that human aspirations would allow us to return to that kind of lifestyle. Understandably we want comforts, we want to enjoy our lives, we want to take advantage of the myriad of opportunities and pleasures that technology has brought us.

We are uniquely social beings and as human culture has evolved so has the place that food plays in our social lives. It is now a central part of our interactions and our social structure, both private and communal. Family events are celebrated with special meals, as are national events like Thanksgiving and many religious events. Eating with friends, whether in a restaurant or at a barbecue, is essential to the way we live our social lives. Even funerals are usually followed by a meal for the mourners. And much business is done over a meal—the business lunch appears to be surviving the credit crunch.

An author confesses

One of the features of our contemporary culture is that we now think of obesity as a problem. Many of us want to lose weight and cannot—we find it as hard as a smoker does to change our habits. As Mark Twain remarked about smoking ('It is easy to give it, up—I have done it hundreds of times'), so it is with weight loss. One of the authors of this book has lost about 20 kg three times in his life, getting down to a respectable 75 kg, and each time has put it back on gradually over several months. As he embarks on his fourth attempt he swears that he will succeed this time . . . really? Given that he is particularly well informed on the subject and very clear about the health benefits of reducing his body weight, why is he finding it so difficult? And why does the other author not have such problems—he can eat and drink as much as he likes and yet remain thin. He has never even considered dieting, and is never aware of eating too much. Both of us have equal motivation to be healthy—or maybe just to look good around campus—we both have detailed knowledge of the biology and understand the consequences of being overweight, but we are obviously very different in our ability to regulate our body weight.

Even casual observation will reveal some marked behavioural differences between the two of us. Place a bowl of cashew nuts in front of us as we are typing away here, and Mark will eat a few of them and then lose interest, whereas Peter will nibble and nibble and nibble until none are left. Mark does not need to think about it; Peter has to consciously stop himself from having another handful and he will still probably eat them. Yet Mark may announce in mid-afternoon that he is absolutely ravenous and cannot survive until suppertime unless he has fruit cake for tea. For Peter hunger in the middle of the afternoon is not the issue, and he has to avoid such snacks—because snacking for Peter does not mean one slice of cake: it means all the slices on the plate.

We are clearly very different in our metabolic biology. And it is only through understanding why we have such differences that we will get a broader perspective on why simple magic bullet strategies—that new diet for example—will not be effective in assisting or sustaining weight loss for most individuals. By the same reasoning, one standard approach is not going to deal with the burden of diabetes and cardiovascular disease in different individuals and across populations. We would go further—we believe that unless we understand the biology of the problem better we have little hope of getting to the right solution to the problem at all. This is one of the key messages of this book.

The simple answer

This is an inconvenient truth (as Al Gore called his film on global warming, and for somewhat similar reasons) for many governments, public health organizations and individual experts who want to treat or prevent obesity, diabetes, and cardiovascular disease with a simple single remedy. They seem to believe that there is a magic bullet which will solve the problem. This is illogical and it will not work. Ban sugary soft drinks, they say, or ban the use of trans-fats in prepared foods, or ban butter, or make the fast food chains reduce their portion sizes, etc., and there will be no problem.

There is a political dimension here because the debate rapidly gets wrapped up with issues of our individual rights to make choices versus the business of the State in controlling our lives. There are those who believe the State has no business to intervene in matters of personal choice, and others who expect the State to play a major role in managing our lives. The debate can be between extremes or it can be a matter of degree. Few people would disagree with the State demanding that we wear seat belts in our cars, or that motorcyclists wear safety helmets. It is clear that in doing so the State is helping us, for our own good, but it probably also reduces the cost to the State and to us all if there is an accident. Some countries require that children are vaccinated before going to school, while others do not, and issues of personal choice—here on the part of the parents—underlie that debate too. And so it goes on. Should the State require you to have energy-saving light bulbs in your house or is it none of their business? Should the State require you to have social security or health insurance? These debates of individual freedom versus State influence rage in different ways in every democracy. Only the issues vary across the world.

Smoke and mirrors

Let us use smoking as an example. The evidence that smoking harms our health is now 50 years old. Yet it took a long time before efforts to reduce smoking were 'owned' by the State. There were vested commercial interests trying to confuse the picture but nicotine addicts also did not want the State limiting their freedom to smoke. They claimed they had the right to make their own choices, even if these harmed their health. But what about passive smoking? It too does harm. This increased the justification for banning smoking. Four things happened more or less simultaneously to put the final nail in the smoking coffin: the industry was vilified by activists; smokers were ostracized; governments started restricting where smoking could be allowed, first on planes, then in restaurants and all public places; and taxes were raised to higher and higher levels on tobacco products—the last has probably been the most effective measure. And although it took many years to implement, the reduced incidence of smoking has clearly improved public health and is a great example of what such a policy can do.

But there is one fundamental difference about smoking—we do not need to do it. We can live without cigarettes and tobacco—after all, Europeans only started smoking tobacco, chewing it, or snorting it about 500 years ago. Yes, it turned into a giant industry and made a lot of people rich and, yes, its tax dollars have appealed to many governments. In China, for example, where there are more than 350 million smokers, who consume one-third of the world's cigarettes smoked every day, 8 per cent of the state revenue comes from tobacco. Its addictive properties are associated with some apparently beneficial psychological effects for many. But its deleterious effects on health far outweigh all this. So once the evidence that it did harm was accepted, and particularly once the evidence that other people's smoke also did harm to non-smokers became clear, the political process of acting to reduce smoking became feasible and is now generally accepted. Plans to ban smoking in public places were put in place in China in 2011 and are starting to be effective.

So would it be logical for state-enforced public health interventions to be introduced to reduce obesity, diabetes, and cardiovascular disease? Superficially it might seem so and the approach has its advocates. But it is based on faulty logic.

Smoking is an indulgence (tobacco) rather than something essential (food, exercise, sleep). If there is a similarity between eating and smoking, it might be that for some people eating too much, and eating unhealthy foods, is an addiction in the same way that smoking is an addiction. There is some limited evidence that nicotine and some types of food can stimulate the same pleasure-producing areas in the brain. This makes make both habits hard to break. But even if obesity were the sign of an addiction—which we generally do not think it is—we have learnt that legislation hardly helps with addiction in many societies. Class A drugs may be illegal but addicts will often do anything, whether legal or not, to get their supply. And surely we do not think that taking insufficient exercise is addictive?

So are we saying that there is nothing that the State should ban or regulate when it comes to food? Hardly. There are some things that would make sense, like banning the advertising of unhealthy foods to young children. But should we ban Coca-Cola because it is basically a sugar load, or foods made with corn oil? Should we try to regulate portion sizes in fast food outlets? If we do any of this do we have to have clear scientific justification, and to be certain that there is no downside? It seems clear to us that there is no downside to banning advertising of certain foods targeted at children – the issue is how to define such foods and, we suspect for reasons that will become clear as this book proceeds, it may well not have as much impact as we would hope. We also see little nutritional justification for consuming soft drinks, but we cannot advance an argument that they should be banned from sale to everyone, because the harmful effect of an occasional soft drink is minimal—the problem is how to encourage people to drink fewer of them.

So the issue we raise is whether measures which might not really make a difference justify interference in our lives and our freedom to choose what we consume. We believe that our attitude to this will also be coloured by our political leaning. The libertarian view would be that it is largely a matter of personal choice. This may be rational if voluntary gluttony and sloth are at the root of the problem. But it becomes more difficult if there are more complex underlying biological factors that make some individuals more or less vulnerable to developing disease in the modern nutritionally rich, technologically dense world. The alternative view might be that the State has the duty to protect us—if necessary, from ourselves.

Why worry?

Before going further we might ask the question—how much do we really need to worry about these issues? Surely, modern medicine will find wonderful treatments for diabetes and cardiovascular disease?

Indeed, once vascular or heart disease is diagnosed, we can use a variety of techniques, both medical and surgical, to keep blood flowing to the coronary arteries which supply the heart muscle. They are very successful and can often return an individual's heart to a healthy state if there is not too much underlying damage. But this is the realm of advanced medicine. Blood pressure lowering pills are not cheap. The surgical opening of the blood vessels supplying the heart costs tens of thousands of dollars. It is unrealistic to imagine that such expensive techniques can be made available to everyone across the world. So if we think about the burden of coronary heart disease at a global level, prevention rather than treatment has to be our priority.

Diabetes is even more complicated to address—with one possible exception, we have no real cure for it; we can only offer lifestyle advice, drugs, and insulin replacement therapy. Moreover, none of the complications of diabetes are easy or cheap to deal with. Once diabetic renal failure sets in, dialysis or a kidney transplant are the only possible options, neither of which is a feasible response to the growing epidemic. There is no treatment for the nerve damage caused by diabetes, or the blindness, and, sadly, limb amputation remains necessary for those with the most advanced diabetic vascular complications.

So what is the exception we mentioned? It is not medical but surgical. In people with obesity, stomach bypass surgery or banding can cure them of their diabetes. But the surprising thing is that this procedure reverses the diabetic state well before it produces any effect through weight loss. We now think that there are hormones made by the lining of the stomach which affect the way that other hormones, and possibly the brain, work to control metabolism. So this aggressive procedure in some way changes the hormonal balance and restores the ability of insulin to work properly. We really do not yet fully understand how this therapy works and it suggests that there is much more about our biology to be found out, which may lead to new ways to intervene.

But stomach banding and gastric bypass procedures are not free of side effects. They can lead to a variety of gastrointestinal problems which the individual then has to live with, and to metabolic complications. But in a case of morbid obesity, particularly where diabetes and cardiovascular disease have set in, surgery is a sensible option. Critically, such procedures seem to reduce fat inside the abdomen, the visceral fat which has the most damaging effects. They also limit the capacity of the intestinal system to absorb fats so that the energy balance is changed. And the reduction in stomach size leads to an earlier sensation of a full stomach during a meal, so the individual eats less.

In gastric banding both the problem of obesity and diabetes and the underlying biology are tackled together. Contrast this with another surgical technique—liposuction. All that the plastic surgeon is doing by sucking out the fat under the skin is providing cosmetic support. The individual may feel that his or her biological problem is being addressed but in reality it is literally only skin deep. The biology driving the obesity remains unchanged. It is no different from using wallpaper to cover the structural defects in a house before it is sold. Sooner or later the problem will appear again.

These two different surgical approaches to obesity raise the question of who should pay the bill. This might depend on whether the surgery is for cosmetic or for medical reasons. It is not always clear, and different medical insurers and governments are struggling with this question. Even if it is certain that the reason is medical, the answer to this question may still be determined by whether we believe that obesity is the individual's own fault, or whether it is understood that for many of us there are deeper underlying biological causes for our obesity.

One of the major problems in discussing overweight and disease is understanding the motivation of the person wanting to undergo weight loss, and the possible psychological and other benefits which might follow the treatment. Is the goal of the treatment related to appearance or to health? The reality is that in the West most attempts at weight loss have more to do with social perception than with health.

The ideal body

The Western ideal body image, particularly for a female, is increasingly about thinness and a particular body shape—an ideal that for most people is neither realistic nor necessarily healthy. There have been many books written on the question of the female body image and the issue is certainly not simple. Contrast the Western ideal with the body image from the areas of Mauritania we discussed earlier, where the ideal body image for a female (or maybe it is for her partner?) is unhealthily obese. We all live within our own societies and cultural networks and in dealing with matters of body size we need to understand these various cultural dynamics.

The psychotherapist Susie Orbach, whose clients have included public figures like Princess Diana, has published books about these issues—*Fat is a Feminist Issue*, which she wrote in 1978, and more recently *Bodies*, about Western women and their bodily concerns. In recent interviews Orbach explained that at the time when *FIFI* (as she likes to call her book) was published, she had no idea that the issue would still be current 30 years later.

In *FIFI*, Orbach argued that overeating in women can be a sign of their unhappiness with their position in society, and also a comfort and something which becomes an end in itself. At one extreme some women might feel that by allowing themselves to become overweight they make themselves less attractive, to men in particular, and therefore remove themselves from the sexual game, distancing themselves from the industry and the media hype focused on thinness. Why spend the week starving yourself so that you can have that magazine-image body and allow yourself to eat only at the weekend with your boyfriend or partner? Why bother—are you really a different person if you gain a few, or even a few dozen, kilograms? Susie Orbach admits that it was her preoccupation with dieting which took her to a self-help group, and it was there that she realized just how deep the hatred of their bodies was among the women who attended the group.

In her later book *Bodies,* Orbach goes on to explore wider issues of the management of the body, from steroid therapy to breast enlargement and other uses of plastic surgery. The theme which concerned her in *FIFI* arises again. No one seems to feel happy with their body as it is, and they feel that they have to work on it—or have work done on it—to spend money, and undergo pain and suffering in order to turn it into the body which should really be theirs—if the advertising is true. Other worries about work, about relationships, about simply getting old and the fear of death become focused on perfecting the body. What has happened naturally cannot possibly be right—there must be some way of correcting it, of improving on it. The fact that it is not right must be the fault of the owner of the body, of his or her laziness or greed or lack of dedication to the cause of perfect beauty.

There is another extremely worrying undercurrent here. The glossy magazines and the media sell images of the idealized bodies of celebrities and glamour models with their perfect pregnancies, giving birth to perfect children, and of course living perfect lives. All this costs an extraordinary amount of money and lesser mortals can only aspire to such a body or such a life. As an actress is supposed to have said some years ago, 'Money does not buy everything, but the other things are so expensive.' And so an industry has grows, built on the conspicuous consumption of what is essentially an artificially constructed fashion.

A generation ago there were wider margins in what was acceptable as the 'ideal' female shape, although thinness has had a premium in the West for a long time (think of Twiggy in the 1960s). Then having the right tan was equally important, and the package holiday industry was built on this myth. Luckily, we now realize the dangers of sunbathing in relation to skin cancer, and so our body image cannot be fixed just by a two-week holiday in the sun. But while most people are more sensible about this aspect of their appearance, we do not seem to have gotten there in relation to obesity.

Social bodies

We cannot get away from considering the social dimension. It seems no accident then that the problems of obesity, diabetes, and cardio-vascular disease are particularly associated with lower socio-economic status in Western societies. This appears to accord with Orbach's idea of disenfranchisement with the values of society, where some people feel that they do not relate to them. But it also makes it clear that the problem is intractable.

Poverty is connected with an unhealthy lifestyle in many ways. For example, when researchers in the UK asked a selection of women how often their family sat down to have a meal together at the table, the question was met with puzzlement from a substantial proportion—as many as 50 per cent in some parts of the country—'Sit round a table? But we don't have a table.' In these households meals are consumed on the sofa in front of the TV, or in bedrooms, or as snacks taken around the house. Clearly this is not likely to be conducive to a balanced diet. Beyond that, the simple and sad reality is that the cheapest foods tend to be least healthy.

There is another possible argument underlying the risks for people in difficult circumstances that emerges from a surprising source, evolutionary biology. Evolution is concerned with success-ful reproduction, not health or longevity. In many animals, when life is threatened, their rate of sexual maturation accelerates so as to ensure reproduction is achieved before death occurs. A respected evolutionary psychologist, Daniel Nettle from Newcastle, has pointed out that this might also be happening in humans. He argues that without a conscious change in behaviour there are evolutionar-ily embedded drivers that lead people in deprived circumstances to hurry up their lives. They reproduce early and more often, they often have earlier puberty, and they make many choices in their lives that suggest they are not investing for the long term.

Unhealthy eating and storing excess energy now for threatening times later could well be part of an evolutionarily determined strategy to anticipate a difficult life-course. Similarly, the motivation to invest in lifestyle choices which only give a delayed advantage in the form of better health later would not be a logical strategy if life is expected to be short. There is no way of evaluating such a hypothesis and we really do not know to what extent unconscious human behaviour is informed by evolutionary echoes. But in other domains of understanding human behaviour and psychological health, the evolutionary perspective has been quite informative.

There are several critical factors that determine whether a family consumes a healthy diet. Firstly, they have to have the knowledge of what such a diet comprises. We will return to this in more detail elsewhere in the book. Secondly, they must have access to the components of such a diet, and lastly, they must have the funds to buy them. Looking at the situation of many families in the more deprived areas of cities in the developed world, we see immediately that none of these three conditions are likely to be met. The members of the family who make the decisions about what food they eat are very often not those who are best informed. Frequently, it is the children or the male head of the household who makes these decisions, and surveys have shown just how badly informed these individuals can be when it comes to nutrition.

Then if we look in the corner shops or small retail outlets which provide the basic necessities in such parts of our cities we find that they seldom provide much in the way of fresh fruit and vegetables, fish, brown bread, etc. All these items are just too perishable and too costly to bring to the shop in small quantities. So it turns out that the healthiness of a diet consumed by a family is very closely linked to how far they live from a major supermarket, whether they have transportation, and so on.

Finally, the reality is that healthy food is relatively expensive compared to junk food, or at least it is thought to be so. True, with skill, care, and patience it is possible to make very healthy meals cheaply from simple ingredients, but all this takes just that—training and time—and these are often in short supply. In fact, lack of time is the most common excuse given by a range of adults for not engaging in much physical exercise, and yet the average person in the UK spends 30 hours a week watching television.

The strange case of Japan

The issue is not only associated with poverty, however, because the choice to eat an inadequate diet can be quite culturally specific. In Japan, there has been a shift in the ideal body image. In the past, as in other Asian societies, a degree of plumpness was seen as a sign of a healthy, potentially fertile woman, one eligible for marriage. But as Western culture has invaded and replaced aspects of traditional culture, many young women have become obsessed with their body image and try desperately to lose weight to look like supermodels. This is made easier because the Japanese diet is traditionally low in carbohydrates, including sugars, and in fat. Additionally, an increasing number of young Japanese women are beginning to smoke. Smoking does not really suppress appetite, as is often believed, but it gives us something to do at a tea break at the office or when we feel in need of comfort.

So many Japanese women, especially in cities, tend to be thinner than would have been 'desirable' in past generations. But they should put on weight during pregnancy, shouldn't they? Ideally, yes, but it turns out that many of them do not gain sufficient weight during pregnancy to support the optimal growth of their baby. Many obstetricians in Japan recommend only a low level of weight gain in pregnancy, even in women who are already extremely thin. Why?

The idea appears to have originated from an over-interpretation of studies of women who became pregnant during a famine in the Netherlands during the latter part of the Second World War. This famine, known as the Dutch Hunger Winter, occurred when the Nazis imposed severe rationing on the Dutch population of the western Netherlands in reprisal for resistance activities. The famine lasted from late 1944 until the Allies liberated the Netherlands in 1945. Because good medical records were kept in some hospitals in the Netherlands despite the circumstances, these women and their children—and now even their grandchildren—have been the subject of detailed investigation of the long-term effects of famine during pregnancy.

The Dutch Hunger Winter studies have produced some unique data which have been very influential in showing the importance of fetal development to the risk of later developing chronic disease, an important concept which we will discuss in Chapter 7. But for some reason Japanese obstetricians focused on an idea, apparently derived from these studies but for which there is essentially no evidence, that eating very little in the first third of pregnancy protects the woman against the potentially dangerous disease of pregnancy, pre-eclampsia. Somehow this unsubstantiated idea migrated to Japan (although nowhere else), and obstetricians there began to advise women to restrict their weight gain in pregnancy. This has done nothing to prevent or reduce the risk of pre-eclampsia, but it has led to Japan being the only country in the developed world where average birth weight has fallen over the past two decades, especially in the major cities. The effect is surprisingly large—the average birth weight has fallen by almost 200 g in that time and, as we shall see later, this may have very important consequences for those people born at this time.

We can see here an all too familiar pattern where a coincidence of events and ideas conspires to produce a bad effect. This was another 'perfect storm'—an idea from older studies which had never been properly substantiated, coupled with doctors deciding as a community to take action to prevent a particularly debilitating disease, plus women's obsession with their body image in the late 20th century— and all this was happening in a population where, by and large, people adhere to the advice which they are given.

Finally, the women themselves were not likely to be concerned about this issue. In many cultures, it is believed that having a small baby is less risky for both mother and baby during labour. There is even a Japanese proverb which says, 'It is better to start small and then grow big.' As we will see later, this may not be such good advice.

Politically incorrect

While we were finishing this book a report from the Organisation for Economic Co-operation and Development (OECD) appeared. The 34 countries represented in the OECD range from the USA to Slovenia, from Norway to Chile. The Commission of the European Community also took part in the work which led to the report. The report is 265 pages and represents the work of many years of research and consultation. It contains the results of very detailed economic modelling of the cost-benefit ratio of various interventions, trying to put a price on non-communicable disease and to determine the economic value of some initiatives, such as educational ones, and weighing them against the likely savings for society in terms of reducing the cost of disease.

The authors of this report have arrived at some apparently definition conclusions. One is that the most effective way of reducing the burden of obesity in adults is to arrange for them to have repeated consultations with a health professional to keep them up to the mark with their diet and exercise programmes. However, this is also a very expensive intervention and cannot be made widely available even in developed, let alone developing, societies. The report—as with others like it, although we have to say that this is an extreme example—hardly refers to the variation between people in their propensity to become obese or to lose weight, and no consideration is given to how differences in metabolism between people develop. Sadly, it appears to have been written without consideration of the reality of human variation and biology.

And recent reports from the World Health Organization do not do much better. Indeed it is extraordinary how many of the so-called experts on the problem seem to ignore the science underlying the problems and go straight to their favourite solution, which is always familiar. It is the same old tale: give humans the chance and they will all be guilty of the sins of gluttony and sloth, with the consequences of obesity, diabetes, and cardiovascular disease—end of story. But, as we shall see, it is not.

We were concerned to read in the OECD report that the determinants of obesity divide into three components. The first are supply-side factors—by which the authors of the report mean the food industry, advertising, and production techniques for highly processed foods. Secondly, there are government policies including those on public transport, taxation, and the provision of recreational facilities for exercise. And thirdly, there are changes in working conditions that lead to reduced physical labour and higher stress levels. Where is the biological perspective here? It is missing. The approach is like trying to solve the problem of why your car will not start without knowing about starter motors and fuel pumps and batteries—but insisting that there must be a problem with the key. Throughout the report, which goes into quite sophisticated socio-economic analysis, the underlying belief is that people who don't eat excessive amounts of unhealthy foods and who undertake regular physical exercise don't usually get very fat. *Therefore* the answer to the problem of obesity is to prevent people from over-indulging themselves and to make them exercise. Nowhere is the possibility even considered that this is not strictly logical and that the truth might be somewhat more complex.

Public opinion and politics

How we respond as individuals to a changing world and to our morphing body shapes is not straightforward. Despite the apparent simplicity of the energy equation, dieting and exercise do not solve the problem because many people are unable to lose much weight, or if they lose weight they soon put it back on. Furthermore, motivations vary between societies because perceptions of body shape are very different across cultures and genders, and are influenced by circumstances.

We need to conclude this chapter by thinking more about public opinion and the politics of obesity, diabetes, and cardiovascular disease. To illustrate the argument, it is worth returning to the public health anti-smoking initiative. Research has shown that the reduction in smoking in some parts of the population has been heavily influenced by taxation, and by legislation to ban smoking in public places. But while these measures have been enormously helpful, they have been politically possible only because of another motivation. And that motivation is stigmatization.

Society has vilified the smoker, and smoking in public has become 'unacceptable' behaviour. Humans evolved to live in social groups and no one can live comfortably within a group where they suffer social approbation. That is why smoking in Western countries is now confined largely to groups such as adolescents, who are used to challenging social norms and facing potential approbation—they want to be seen as outlaws and rebels. This is probably more true of young men, but young women too are increasingly likely to smoke, especially in parts of the developing world where the tobacco industry is specifically targeting advertising at them.

We worry that there is a growing tendency among some public health practitioners to adopt a similar strategy with respect to obesity—that is to stigmatize those who are obese and to vilify the food industry or try to ban certain food components. Some commentaries are adopting an increasingly shrill tone, declaring that the problem is all about fructose or all about trans-fats or all about vitamins. It is suggested that a simple ban like that on smoking could work. Ban McDonald's and all will be well. Ban soft drinks and all will be well. There are many reasons why this will fail—and at the end of the campaign the very people who need most assistance will still be obese and at still greater risk of disease.

Any solution will be somewhat complex. We have a pipeline of food supplies that is very different from that of our ancestors. Food is now not simple—increasingly, our diet is not what comes out of the ground, off the tree, or from an animal. More and more foods are manufactured from extensively processed ingredients, loaded with additives, and having undergone chemical changes. The mixture of fats and carbohydrates we consume and our sources of protein are very different from what they once were. And more changes take place all the time, given the power and size of the food industry on the one hand and the way we want to live our lives on the other. Before television came along we had no need for TV meals—do we really need them now? Not really, but we like the convenience.

Our argument is that, if we are to tackle the problem of obesity, diabetes, and cardiovascular disease effectively, several parts of the equation are missing. We will discuss other gaps later but an important one is quite simply, knowledge. Hardly anyone, wherever they live, has a real understanding of what they are eating and what they should eat. The pace of change in the nature of the food supply and the way we live our lives means that for many people traditional family-based knowledge about food is insufficient. The food our parents bought (or grew) and the way that they cooked and served it bear little relation to our food pipeline today. And we have already seen how poor eating and other lifestyle habits can run in families, so leaving the imparting of knowledge about healthy nutrition only to parents is more likely to reinforce disadvantage in those who do not consume a good diet now.

Quite clearly, governments need to insist that knowledge about healthy eating is included in the school curriculum, and even the preschool curriculum, for data show that nutritional education at an early age can have long-lasting effects. It is irresponsible and inadequate to delegate this job to parents who are often not prepared to take on this task. In addition, there is increasing evidence that teaching children about good nutrition influences the eating habits of the whole family.

But some politicians insist that the State should not be involved in these matters. They see it rather as sex education used to be viewed— as something personal and private that should be left entirely to parents to impart to their children. The battle for sex education has been won, at least in many developed countries (although some schools still leave it until it is too late). We argue vehemently that in the same way it is totally unrealistic to rely on nutritional information and lifestyle skills being transmitted from parent to child. Many—possibly most—parents do not know the facts, and given the speed of change in nutrition they are not in a position to do anything to change the situation.

Education means genuine knowledge about what food contains, and about what healthy and unhealthy eating are. It is about the energy equation and the consequences of unbalanced diets and the lack of physical exercise. It is also important to avoid all the misinformation that tends to creep into nutritional information, for example overzealous health claims for antioxidants or misleading claims about some food types. Educational information must be accurate. This is similar to the case for genetically modified foods. There may be other reasons, some largely value-laden, why people do not want to eat such foods, but the claims that those opposed to them make regarding their safety are generally unscientific or totally exaggerated.

And then there is the problem of the food label. Many countries now require packaged foods to be labelled. But there is enormous variation in what is required and most of the information is dense, and effectively meaningless. It is expressed in terms that a nutritional scientist, let alone a consumer, can barely understand and so cannot be of much help. We need to provide simple, clear information against the background of the education needed to understand it. Knowing that 100 g of a food contains 12 per cent of the recommended daily allowance of niacin is meaningless and useless information. What does the recommended daily allowance mean and, in any event, how does 100 g relate to what is being eaten? In any case, there are very few people who need to know how much niacin they are eating.

What we need to know exactly is how much energy is in our food and what form it takes. And we need to know how many calories a day we should eat. We have asked professional people who are not doctors or nutritionists this question and been shocked at the variation in answers we have received—from a few hundred to 5,000 calories a day. If university graduates do not know the answer to this basic question, nutritional literacy is a real problem. In New York, fast food outlets now have to show how many calories are in their hamburgers. Given that fast food is a main source of meals for so many people, this is welcome, but again if we do not know how many calories we should eat each day, does it really help to know if one burger has 550 or 1,550 calories?

Blame the food industry

If the obese person or family is one target for zealous interventions, another is the food industry itself. It is easy to rail against this industry, but in reality not only does it influence what we want but it also sells us what we want. This is complex because fatty foods tend to be tastier—many taste-evoking substances are dissolved in fat—and in many cases they are cheaper to make and have a longer shelf life. We buy them because we like them, they are cheap, and they keep—we are not being totally exploited here. Mind you, the industry has had its knuckles rapped, justifiably, for making excessive claims about the health benefits of some foods and for fast food advertising targeted at children.

But on the other hand, without the food industry the capacity of the world to support seven billion people—let alone the nine or ten billion people we expect—is doubtful. The food industry is a necessary part of every economy, from the poorest to the richest country.

Food security is an urgent concern for many governments. Supplying food to a hungry world requires the involvement of the private sector. We need their cooperation. We need them to produce healthier foods and to restrict their profit-driven emphasis on producing unhealthy foods. The issue is how much carrot and how much stick we should use. There will be a place for restricting some activities, such as marketing junk food to children—but how do we define junk food? And equally we need the food industry to be our partner in finding a way to produce cheap, healthy food. Getting the balance right requires open minds and a willingness to engage in a partnership rather than a fight.

We urgently need a constructive engagement with that industry to find ways in which they can profit and we can live healthily. Denying this is as illogical as saying that we will not encourage car manufacturers to make safer cars, because when they sell them to us they make a profit from our safety. Safer cars are in our mutual interest.

Earlier in this chapter we stressed that we are all different, in terms of our metabolism, our appetites and tastes, as well as our self-control. Mark can resist the bowl of cashew nuts; Peter cannot. Some people can be fat but not at great risk of diabetes or cardiovascular disease; others seem to be relatively thin but have problems of excess visceral fat and a greatly increased risk of such disease. We need to understand these differences—how much are they due to genetic differences, how much are they population-based, and how much are they due to personal, cultural, and biological factors? For until we do so we cannot appreciate when it is appropriate to tackle the issue of obesity and chronic disease prevention at a population level and when to tackle it on an individual basis. Until then we cannot make real progress—so this is where we need to go next.

6

Genes Aren't Us

The hunt for the genes

Each of us responds differently to living in the modern world. One of the great achievements of Charles Darwin was the recognition that individual variation matters. In what he called natural selection, he described how some variations make an individual more likely to survive and reproduce and others less likely to do so. When such variation was inherited, partly through what we now call genes, those who reproduced most successfully left more descendants, who in turn had more favourable genetic endowments than those who reproduced less successfully. This process gradually changes the population over generations, so that the characteristics of most of its individuals match the environment they inhabit. This is as true for bees and trees as it is for animals, including humans.

The implications of this for understanding modern humans are important. Evolution is generally a gradual process. Real change in what makes us what we are by this process takes many generations.

But only a few generations have passed since a big change in our world took place with the industrial revolution. And there have been surprisingly few generations since we invented agriculture and started settling in villages and then in larger towns and cities. Most of human evolution had already happened in Africa. When we look at our history in this way we can readily understand that our biology is largely designed by evolution for a very different world from the one we inhabit today.

But Darwin recognized that the 'survival of the fittest' was not the only way in which genetic variation could influence a population. Many animals also choose their mates. The choice in many species is made by a female, who decides which male she prefers. This is common in birds, and it is often said that this is why male birds evolved with some particularly attractive characteristics — at least to female birds. These might be the colour of their feathers (males tend to be the more colourful sex), how they sing (only male songbirds sing), how they make a bower, a particular kind of courtship dance, or the length of their feathers (think of peacocks). In many mammals the males fight or compete for mating rights with the female. So the gorilla defends his harem until he is displaced by another male; the elk fights with other male elk for dominance of the herd; the bull elephant seal spends much of his time on the beach fighting off other males. Darwin called this kind of process sexual selection.

Both natural and sexual selection are based on variation in our genes—in other words it was not what made us all the same that was important, but what made each of us different. We each have about 21,000 different genes and every cell in our body has the same set. Genes are made of DNA and it is the DNA that forms our chromosomes.

But although all humans basically have the same repertoire of genes, we may vary in the number of copies of these genes we have and in their detailed structure. Each gene contains thousands of connected molecules of DNA, subunits called nucleotides. It is the sequence of these nucleotides that creates the particular gene and provides the genetic instructions which make our bodies work. Genes operate by instructing cells to make proteins such as enzymes, hormones, and the structural components that hold our body together. But these nucleotide sequences can have subtle variations between individuals, and that variation is reflected in the way we each have a slightly different genetic repertoire. It turns out that there is actually an extraordinary amount of subtle variation between individuals.

Each chromosome is made up of a long chain of DNA which thus comprises about 1,000 genes. But each gene on a chromosome is separated by sections of DNA which are not active genes. Indeed most of the DNA on a chromosome is not part of any gene. This used to be called 'junk' DNA but one of the most exciting developments in molecular biology has been the discovery that this DNA functions to control the switches which instruct the genes when to be turned on and off. Much of the variation in DNA structure lies in these control regions, which leads to even more subtle variation in gene function between individuals.

So do genes explain why we respond differently to living in a world of plenty? In the early 1960s the geneticist James Neel was pondering the question of why the Pima Indians living in Arizona, whom we introduced in the last chapter, showed such a high level of diabetes. Many young adults were clearly insulin-resistant (the technical way of describing the condition when insulin does not work properly in tissues such as our muscles), a condition that is the forerunner of diabetes. Some Pima had even developed diabetes in their thirties. Neel wondered whether the Pima had a genetic predisposition to the disease, and if so, why it occurred in this population in particular, rather than in others. When he thought about the history of these native American people, living for centuries on subsistence agriculture in their tribal homeland, he wondered if their evolutionary history might have contributed to the phenomenon.

Could it be, Neel wondered, that over the course of many generations this particular isolated population had undergone natural selection and become well adapted to their harsh nutritional conditions? If so, might it be that genes which conferred an advantage under these conditions had been selected? He called such possible genes 'thrifty' and suggested that they might be genes which conferred a level of insulin resistance in the body. After all, if insulin does not work as well as it should, metabolically active tissues such as skeletal muscle take up less glucose. This means that the body runs on less of this fuel, a bit like a car engine set to run on a leaner rather than a richer mixture of fuel and air. Indeed the Pima Indians were lean or at least had been lean under their traditional way of life.

But then many Pima changed their way of life, particularly in Arizona. This change came in the form of soft drinks and hamburgers and fries, which were widely available along with ice cream, doughnuts, and chocolate chip cookies, as well as alcohol. The Pima also took up sedentary jobs and drastically reduced the amount of manual work they undertook. So the people whose metabolism was set to run on a lean setting were now at very high risk. Here they were, with insulin not working properly, saturating their bodies with sugar and fat from their diet. Needless to say, the calories which could not now be used by muscle were stored as fat. Neel believed that all this was due to the Pima having a different genetic repertoire. His argument seemed highly plausible and was extremely influential. Perhaps these Indians had provided us with a vital clue—if the genes that caused them to have diabetes could be found, then we might know why many of us also get diabetes. This spawned a generation of medical research activity to find the thrifty genes.

But problems were soon found with the story. There was no dispute that thrifty metabolism might lead to metabolic problems, including obesity, diabetes, and cardiovascular disease, in a rich environment—but could the genes be found? A lot of studies looked for gene variations to explain the findings but the data were rather unconvincing. Only a small amount of disease risk could be explained by the gene differences found. And when it was pointed out that those Pima Indians still living in Mexico had a much lower incidence of diabetes although they were genetically very similar to the Arizonan Pima, the genetic explanation seemed harder to sustain. Indeed the Mexican Pima had an incidence of diabetes very similar to other ethnic groups living near them, but who were very different genetically, suggesting that there was no added genetic risk. It appeared that environment, far more than genes, was influencing the occurrence of diabetes in the Arizonan Pima.

This example concerns a rather specific group of people living in a particular part of the world. What about the general population of a country like the UK or the USA? There is large variation in obesity levels and the risk of getting diabetes, so if genetic explanations were responsible, we would also expect there to be large differences in genetic make-up.

The understanding that there were many small differences in the structure of genes between people led to the search for associations between these differences and a high risk of disease. The concept became simplified to the idea that there might be genes 'for' certain conditions such as diabetes, obesity, or high blood pressure, when what was really being meant was that there were particular structural changes in genes that led to greater disease risk. In the 1990s immense amounts of research dollars were ploughed into the Human Genome Project to build on this very idea. If only, the scientists argued, we knew the complete structure of the human genome, all the sequence of the nucleotides in the DNA strands that make up our chromosomes and which provide the code for developing a human being, we might be able to find the particular regions where small differences between individuals change disease risk.

These small differences in an individual's genetic make-up are called polymorphisms. Because they are found in the genetic material, they are likely to be passed from mother and father to son and daughter, along lines of inheritance. The search for genes 'for' disease depended on having a dictionary of all the genes in the human genome. Compiling that dictionary became a race between a publicly funded consortium in the UK and in Washington and the private enterprise of Craig Venter in the USA. After an enormous amount of pioneering work, and with a great fanfare, the human genome sequence was published almost simultaneously by these two independent endeavours.

Now the fun really started. Where were the gene variants that explained cardiovascular disease or diabetes? Some genes were found that were associated with obesity. An example was the FTO gene (the researchers involved apparently wondered whether to call it the FATSO gene but thought better of it). People who have one particular variant of the FTO gene have a higher chance of becoming fat. Great! The concept of the thrifty gene or the fat gene was proven. Or was it? Well, not quite, because while it is true that people with this particular polymorphism are at greater risk of becoming fat, the reverse is not true. The vast majority of people who become fat do not have this polymorphism in their FTO gene. All cats are animals, but not all animals are cats. In fact the FTO polymorphism did not explain much of the obesity pattern at all.

So the search continued. More gene candidates turned up where variations in the gene sequence were associated with some increase in the risk of obesity, but the degree of added risk they conferred and the amount of obesity they explained were generally rather small. By now there about two dozen genes clearly linked to obesity but the amount of fatness in the population that these variants explain still remains small. Indeed, even taking all these genes into account identifies less than 10 per cent of the people in a Western population who become fat. The conclusion must be that genes do not hold the answer—well, at least, inherited polymorphisms are not the answer. Some researchers have argued that the problem is an analytical one and we need more sophisticated techniques, but only a relatively small fraction of obesity and disease risk—perhaps a quarter—can be explained by using even the most optimistic estimates.

And then other forms of genetic variation were found. One of the surprises of the Human Genome Project was the discovery that our genetic material varies more than expected because some of us carry multiple copies of some genes. This so-called copy number variation was then studied to see if it could provide the genetic link to disease risk that polymorphisms had not. Again small effects were seen, and again, in terms of explaining the variation in disease risk, the results were disappointing.

This was depressing for the genetic research community, although from a medical point of view we could see it as encouraging. After all, if it had turned out that our risk of being fat versus staying slim was something primarily inherited from our parents as fixed genetic variation, and thus determined inexorably at conception, we would have to take a very deterministic and fatalistic view of life. It would mean that while we could identify those children at birth who would most probably become fat, there would be little we could do about it. We can't re-engineer the human genome in a particular individual. Forget the ideas of gene therapy which have largely turned out to be ineffective, even for diseases where a defect in only one single gene operates, such as cystic fibrosis. For a disorder such as obesity, where a large number of genes might be involved, gene therapy approaches are implausible.

So it was gradually acknowledged that the strong genetic determinism which had driven much of biomedical research for two decades was not particularly helpful in understanding the human condition. Indeed, with only 21,000 genes to explain all our body functions, layers of additional biological control remain to be discovered, and exploring them is a most exciting part of the next generation of scientific enquiries. The complexity of control of gene switches is extraordinary and every year more layers are being uncovered. It is an exciting story to which we will return in the latter part of the book.

The limits of the genes

While the Human Genome Project was a technical and scientific *tour de force*, it did not provide the answers that its most earnest protagonists had hoped for and in intellectual terms it brought with it many problems. Why was this? Part of the problem lay in the mindset of the scientists doing the work and the media which covered them. We still see it operating today, in claims that a gene 'for schizophrenia' or a gene 'for breast cancer' has at last been found. There are of course no such genes because these diseases are complex. Our genes have evolved over time to generate biological control over our development and function. They do very prosaic things in controlling the making of proteins and the function of other genes—the design of our bodies has been refined through the Darwinian selection of these very fundamental functions. Virtually all bodily functions involve many genes acting together, and many genes have multiple forms and functions. All of them operate through complex control processes about which we are still learning. So it is naive to imagine that there would be one gene that causes a particular disease.

Indeed even the concept of a gene is changing. We used to think that genes had only one role—to be the template for proteins to be made, so we identified genes by the proteins for which they coded—the FTO gene made the FTO protein, and so on. That template involves DNA being read, which in turn leads to the production of an intermediary called RNA. Like DNA, RNA is also made of nucleotides. It is the RNA that then gets read by the cell's machinery, which leads to amino acids being joined together to make proteins. But now we know that most RNA made on instruction from DNA does not act to make proteins at all, but rather acts to control gene function itself. These non-coding RNAs (so called because they do not code for proteins) create new levels of molecular control—they represent an exciting new area of biology in which new discoveries emerge every week.

As so often in science, part of the problem lies in our use of words. Genes do not cause disease, but paradoxically we tend to name them after the diseases we identify when an abnormality of a gene leads to disease. So the cystic fibrosis gene is named after the disease that occurs when one particular gene is mutated, but in reality that gene's function is to regulate the amount of chloride going in and out of cells by making a protein which acts as a chloride channel across the cell membrane. It is the malfunction of that channel, caused by a mutation in the gene, that leads to the disease cystic fibrosis. It has been this misuse of genetic deterministic language in talking about genes 'for' a disease that has limited the thinking of many scientists. And cystic fibrosis is a straight-forward example in that it is a very common and well-documented purely genetic disease which occurs only if both the mother and father of the affected child carry a mutated copy of this gene.

But in the chronic disease story, there is no simple genetic pattern to justify a belief in a strong genetic basis. Certainly some genetic vari-ation across a number of genes plays some role in generating greater disease risk, but not that much and we have not been able to find genetic variation of a type that can account for the common occur-rence of obesity and the non-communicable diseases.

Even the 'thrifty gene' concept with which we started this chapter turns out to have a flaw. Neel thought that our Palaeolithic ancestors would have been exposed to cycles of feast and famine and that this would have favoured the survival of individuals who could better lay down fat because they had thrifty genes. In fact there is little evidence that our hunter-gatherer forebears did experience such cycles—they probably moved when food sources became low. Skeletal remains do not suggest that our earliest ancestors suffered greatly from malnutrition.

Furthermore, humans have lived in many different environments over many generations. We are a generalist species, good at respond-ing to changes in environments, and it is probably our ability to use technology to stabilize our environment through, for example, making clothes and shelter and fire which has given us a major advantage over other species on the planet. If we could change the environment, we did not need to change our biology. So trying to find the environment in which our genes are best 'fitted' is wrong, because neither that environment nor a particular set of genes suited to it exists.

Yet we cannot ignore genes completely, for they are important in another sense. Selective mechanisms can only operate across the range of environments our predecessors have been exposed to. For example, if none of our ancestors had been exposed to a particular toxin, whether from a plant or a parasite or a new pesticide, we could not possibly have evolved the genes needed for the detoxifying mechanisms to deal with it. Indeed there are some foods that some species eat with impunity, because they have evolved with the right detoxification mechanism, while they are deadly for other species. For example, there are many berries which are poisonous for humans but which some birds can eat. The differences between the species in this respect are usually genetic, and presumably the genetic basis for the detoxification process has evolved in one species and not another because it was necessary for the former to make use of that food source.

In the same way, it is fairly certain that our ancestors were never exposed to the kind of nutritional levels we now have—they would not have had access to highly refined foods and they did not consume energy-dense diets over prolonged periods of time. The processes of selection that operated on our ancestors could only ensure that their metabolic capacities matched the nutritional intakes of their time. So from an evolutionary perspective the nutritional environments we now confront are essentially entirely novel and we cannot expect to have the genetic repertoire to cope with them.

Until perhaps only 100 years ago, not many of our ancestors would have faced high nutritional loads consistently and continuously. Thus we have evolved with a limit to our capacity to cope with modern energy-dense diets—a limit that we are now increasingly likely to exceed. These concepts of evolutionary novelty and the limits in our evolved capacity to adapt are important because they explain the inevitability of the non-communicable disease epidemic in a world where food supplies have changed so dramatically and so quickly. Because evolutionary processes on the genes are slow, there is no way that we can evolve now to cope with this new nutritional environment. We need to look beyond the gene.

Way beyond our genes

Genetic variation is not the only way in which people differ. They differ in the way they grow up, how they learn, what they are taught, and what they observe. That is why New Zealanders speak English (although the authors disagree on this point) and Brazilians speak Portuguese. That is why orthodox Jews do not eat pork and devout Hindus do not eat beef. That is why some people can swim or fly-fish and some cannot.

What we are is not only a function of our genes. It is a function of the environment we live in, our families, our society, our culture, our physical world. A young woman in rural Mauritania is more likely to be obese than one in Japan for reasons that are embedded in her culture, rather than her genes. A yak herder in Tibet is likely to have to eat much more each day to meet his basic energetic needs than a desk jockey in Hong Kong. And, just as individuals vary in their propensity to get fat or to suffer from a chronic disease, so do populations—and for very much the same reasons.

Populations inhabit and create very different environments: the experiences of a child in northern California are likely to be very different from those of a child in Ethiopia. One will be more likely to have had a well-nourished and healthy mother, a safe birth, good nutrition and immunization in infancy, as well as an education, but at the same time to have been exposed to excess amounts of energy-dense foods and to have spent much of their time in front of a TV screen. Populations clearly also vary in their economic status, in family structures, and in the types of exercise they habitually undertake. One child may go out with friends to play a ball game. The other may have the role in the family of bringing 50 litres of water from the river a kilometre away each day.

We can summarize the problem we have been discussing by looking at a famous study by Paul McKeigue and colleagues, published in the early 1990s. McKeigue's group related the waist–hip ratio, which is a good measure of the level of abdominal obesity, to the occurrence of diabetes in different population groups living in the UK. For white Europeans of Caucasian extraction the risk of diabetes for those with a ratio of waist circumference to hip circumference of 1 was about 10 per cent. However, for people of South Asian origin, many of whom had come from the Indian subcontinent early in their lives or in the previous generation, the incidence of diabetes for those with a waist–hip ratio of 1 was about 25 per cent. And at any higher waist–hip ratio, South Asians had about three times the risk of developing diabetes. Of course there are well-known differences in dietary habits between these groups, as well as differences in levels of physical activity and recreational pursuits. If this were the main cause of the difference, then dieting and exercise should be more effective in reducing diabetes in South Asians than in Caucasians, but this is not the case. So is the difference genetic? While some genetic differences clearly exist between the populations, these do not appear to explain the differences in susceptibility to diabetes. Is it because South Asian babies start their lives in a very different way? There are hints that this might be so—these babies are on average smaller at birth than Caucasian babies. We will soon come back to this possibility.

Whatever the explanation, variation between individuals and across populations clearly matters a great deal. Consider two people given precisely the same rations to eat day after day—let's say that they are prisoners in a gaol and are offered a fairly standard set of foods every day. Depending on their genetic make-up, their developmental history, their upbringing, and the context of where they are they could respond very differently. They might differ in their appetite control, so that one eats more than the other. One might have an allergy to a certain component of the diet, say fish, and avoid eating it. Or they might both eat the same amount but because of their biochemical make-up one is more likely to put on fat than the other. Or they might put on the same amount of fat, but one might deposit it under the skin and the other in the liver. Or one might have a strong family history of heart disease and the other might have parents and grandparents who lived until they were 100. Or one might exercise while the other is an invalid. We could go on . . . but it is clear that to predict what will happen to the two individuals exposed to the same dietary regime is not easy. We need to understand all these causes of variation, not just the genes of our two prisoners—and our list is by no means complete.

Medical arts

Many doctors will admit that clinical medicine is as much an art as a science. Historically the practice of medicine, growing as it did from the traditions of the barber surgeons and the apothecaries of the 16th century, has not always had a strictly scientific basis. Only 200 years ago, blood-letting by cupping or using leeches was a common practice to relieve certain 'humours'. However, in the past few decades medical research has exploded. We now know so much more about our biology and the origins of disease, at least in theory. But the diffusion of this new knowledge into medical practice is often much slower. There are many reasons for this. Much biomedical research is highly technical and inaccessible even to doctors. Then the 'art of medicine', something they learn from their teachers and acquire through experience during their careers, leaves individual doctors with their biases. These biases may include the use of alternative medicines such as homeopathy, even when there is no objective evidence that they work and much scientific argument for why they can only have a placebo effect. As one wit put it recently: 'What do you call an alternative medicine for which there is evidence that it works? Orthodox medicine.' This is not to dismiss alternative medicine out of hand—after all, many modern medicines are derived from natural products.

So the level of objectivity in a doctor's choice of what to do may not be as high as is generally thought. This is why one doctor favours one approach to management and is insistent that it is the best approach, while another will vehemently argue for another approach. Often they are both correct—or both wrong—and more often than not the evidence which they need to decide on the course of treatment is missing, not compelling, or hard to access. However, the move towards so-called evidence-based medicine in recent years has been an attempt to systematize what we know and what we do not know, which has gained much support. Large institutes and databases have been established to undertake this type of synthesis. These databases are very useful in describing the general response to a particular therapy, but their limitation is that they treat every individual with the disease as *typical*. And so the new art of medicine is knowing when to apply such averaged approaches to a patient and when not to.

Medicine is in fact a very conservative profession and new knowledge and new paradigms of disease enter its practice very slowly. This contrasts with the rapid development of new technologies such as MRI and CT scanners and the introduction of new drugs. There are inevitable vested interests, which include the influence of drug and equipment companies, insurance companies, hospital administrators, and senior experts in medicine. And increasingly the patient, as an apparently informed determinant of his or her own treatment, influences what the doctor will do; the internet has become empowering in this respect, although most of us are baffled by the sheer amount of information available on any complaint or condition which we feel we might have. Knowing what weight to put on each of such a plethora of 'facts' is where the art lies. That headache, for example—is it a consequence of too much coffee at lunchtime, or is it the first sign of a brain tumour?

The phenomenon of evidence-based medicine has had an important impact. Nowadays young doctors are trained to think in terms of research coming from a range of fields—laboratory investigation, population studies, drug development, and clinical trials. Very often, however, all this evidence does not have an internal consistency and does not provide direct insights into the mechanisms or causes of disease. Rather, what the evidence may do is show that a particular group or subset of the population is more likely to get a particular disease or to respond to a particular treatment. This has been highly successful, for example in establishing the link between smoking and lung cancer, in leading to fluoride being added to the water to prevent to dental caries, and in determining which anti-cancer drug to use for a particular type of tumour.

But even though the evidence from such studies tells us a lot about *when* certain conditions develop, and even perhaps *how* they develop, it does not address the question of *why* they develop. This is a fundamental issue in medicine because it is often difficult to design the most effective treatment if we do not know precisely why the condition has developed. In addition, superficial use of evidence-based approaches implies that all the subjects with a particular disease are similar when, as we have seen with obesity, not everyone is the same.

But how important is the *why* question as opposed to the *when* and *how* questions? Imagine that we are trying to treat people who have high blood pressure. We find something that lowers this pressure— it might be a new drug, it might be a traditional herbal remedy, or it might be a course of yoga or meditation. Does this observation therefore give us the solution for how best to treat high blood pressure in a particular patient? We can see that the answer to this question will be 'it depends ...' It depends, in fact, on many things.

The use of a drug over a long period may be detrimental, either because it produces side effects or because it is too crude in its action. Alcohol consumption will lower blood pressure for a very short period of time, for example, but we would not prescribe a patient regular shots of vodka. What about meditation? It may calm a patient, and if stress was part of their problem it might help to lower their blood pressure—but wouldn't they actually be better spending half an hour each day in the gym rather than sitting cross-legged trying to attain another plane of being? We don't know. And the herbal remedy may work, but how much do we know about its active ingredients? How do such remedies work, and what might be the dangers of sustained use of them? Again, we just don't know.

How do we ever get out of this wood? Are we saying that we can never treat a condition unless we know how the treatment works? Well, almost. This is because the best treatments work through rectifying the problem at its very root, not by just relieving the symptoms. We can stop a patient complaining about the pain from a broken collar bone by giving them morphine, but in the long term it is better to set the fracture. The smartest drugs which we can use to treat the patient with high blood pressure will strike at the cause of the problem by blocking the action of hormones that cause the blood pressure to rise or by preventing the structural changes in blood vessels which make them more rigid. The snag is that to develop such drugs we need to know the causal pathways to the disease in the first place. So we see that knowing why a treatment works is closely bound up with knowing how a disease develops.

Why, oh why?

Why questions can be answered at two levels. The first is at the proximate level—that is the immediate cause question. *Why* does a particular individual have high blood pressure? The proximate answer would be because their blood vessels have been hardened with age and if the heart is pumping a certain amount of blood, the pressure in rigid blood vessels will be higher than it would be if they were flexible. But *why* are the person's blood vessels stiffer? Because most of the elastic tissue in them has been laid down in their early development, before they were born and in infancy, and this tissue becomes less elastic as time goes on. In addition, deposits of calcified fibrous tissue accumulate in the blood vessels throughout life, particularly in response to the inflammatory processes triggered by fats and certain hormones in the bloodstream. But this is still a proximate level answer.

So *why* can be asked again and the answer would be: because it would appear that the human body (and that of many other animals too) has been 'designed' to keep blood pressure and cardiovascular function within a healthy range in the period at least up to the point when a person reproduces, even though this has to be traded off against the decline in function (seen here as arterial stiffness) which in all probability will happen later in life.

This game can become very tedious or annoying, but we can see that we have shifted now to a different level of question—what we can call the ultimate level. Why have the processes of evolution allowed the disease process to exist and why did natural selection not select characteristics which allow us to avoid developing high blood pressure or diabetes? This takes us a long way (and over a long time historically) from modern evidence-based medicine. But it is a journey worth taking.

Evolutionary medicine

The ultimate *why* question brings us to the fundamental principles of a very new field—evolutionary medicine—one we have written about in other books. The processes involved in evolution ultimately operate towards only a single goal—successful reproduction. When the complexities of evolution are peeled away, genetic features which favour successful reproduction are more likely to be passed on to the next generation than those that do not. So over time, in a lineage, the genetic make-up of individuals is increasingly reflected in features that enhance reproduction. In time an equilibrium is reached where the features of the organism are matched well to the environment, provided of course that the environment has not changed.

But when we say 'matched well' we need to interpret this solely in terms of its direct effects on reproduction. A cheetah's coat gives it camouflage in the savannah, its skeletal and muscular structure allow it to run at high speeds, and its sharp teeth and claws allow it to kill its prey. But the reason it is *matched well* is because these are features that allow it to hunt successfully, and better nutrition supports reproduction in the female and gives strength to the male, ensuring reproductive success. Reproductive success plays out in terms of the number of offspring that survive to reproduce themselves.

All of what we have just said is standard evolutionary biology. But the point which is often not recognized is that the drivers of evolution, which protect and enhance effective reproduction, are not always the same ones which might ensure longevity or health. Some species, such as the antichinus family of mouse-like marsupials in Australia, or for that matter the salmon, only reproduce in one season. The male marsupial goes into a mating frenzy and then dies from exhaustion; the male salmon fertilizes thousands of eggs, then also dies. But both have, in their ecological system, maximized their reproductive success and produced lots of offspring. The male praying mantis may even get eaten by his mate as they are in the process of copulation—this changes the meaning of enjoying sex. Health and survival are important for reaching reproductive age, but in general, once reproduction has been completed, there is little advantage—in purely evolutionary terms—in continuing to live. The exception to this rule is in some long-lived but slowly reproducing mammals such as the elephant, or indeed the human. In these there is an advantage in living long enough to ensure that offspring survive to adulthood and themselves reproduce.

Because we usually reproduce before we reach middle age, evolutionary processes operate to maximize survival up to the time of reproduction and are much less concerned with longevity beyond the reproductive period. This has caused the trade-off of biological processes which are designed to favour successful development to reproduction rather than investment in cellular repair and protection mechanisms in later life. This is not an absolute rule, as there is some evidence of a fitness benefit from longevity: for example, the presence of a child's maternal grandmother aids its survival. This 'grandmother effect' may be the origin of the human menopause in that there may be greater evolutionary advantage to a woman assisting her own child to raise children than continuing to reproduce herself, but this is speculative. This effect is relatively weak compared to the selective pressures acting in earlier life, although it might have its echo in women having on average a longer lifespan than men. But in general we have less capacity to cope with challenges to our biology that occur later in life.

It is hard to understand how much modern medicine has changed our perceptions of what to expect of our lives. When Sir William Beveridge set the retirement age for men at 65 in the UK in 1942, their average life expectancy was 62, so less than half of all men would need a pension. At that time much medical care was aimed at addressing the relatively fast decline and demise in adult life—whether from infection or from diseases such as heart disease or cancer, which carried off their victims fairly quickly by today's standards. Treating chronic disease and the demand for a healthy life into the eighth decade or beyond was not then a major focus of attention for most doctors.

We do not know precisely what life expectancy was in our evolutionary past. It is probable that most people had died by the end of the fourth decade of life and relatively few lived to the sixth or seventh decade. Death was largely due to trauma, childbirth, or infection. Reproduction was over by that age so what happened later was of little evolutionary consequence. But now we live on average much longer lives and so disease associated with the failure of repair and maintenance has become more common.

And as we have seen we are living these lives in very different ways, with much greater access to dietary calories and fat. It is this combination of living longer and in different ways that makes it no surprise that modern humans develop various types of chronic disease in middle and older age—indeed, it seems inevitable.

This is all very well but it does not really explain why one person develops a particular type of disease and another does not, even though they appear to live in the same environment and have no other obvious differences. After all, they are both the outcome of the same evolutionary process, aren't they? To understand this we have to address the ultimate *why* question from an ultimate perspective.

A famous demonstration of the power of doing this was the study of growth of children in families who migrated from eastern Europe to the USA in the early 20th century. The distinguished anthropologist Franz Boas made the critical observation that the children who were raised in the USA grew to be several inches taller than their parents, who had grown up in Europe. The same finding has been observed many times—the children of Mayans who had migrated from poor rural Mexico to be, for example, golf course keepers in modern Gainesville, Florida are, within a generation, much taller. What these observations tell us is that our biology, in this case our height, is influenced by more than just our genes. It is influenced by the way we have grown up and in particular by our environment as we were growing up. The parental generation of the eastern Europeans and the Mayans were stunted in childhood by chronic under-nutrition and infection. Their children knew no such constraints.

Let us take an even more telling example. Identical twins have the same genes because they started life when a fertilized egg split into two identical cells. This is a different type of twinning to non-identical twins, when two separate eggs are released in the same menstrual cycle by the mother's ovaries; both are fertilized by two separate sperm, so they have different genetic material. But despite their identical genetic material, identical twins are not really identical. They will not have the same birth weights and in most cases their growth and behaviour and personalities will differ, even if only subtly. But it is when we measure the ways their genes are switched on and off that we see that there are other differences in how their gene control systems are set. These differences accumulate over time after conception so that, as they grow, they become more and more different. These switches will be discussed in more detail in the next chapter but here we only need to say that they are influenced by environmental events which may be experienced by one twin differently from the other. And of course, as they accumulate these genetic switch differences, they are more likely to respond differently even to the same stimulus.

A series of experiments conducted in Canada in the 1990s by the distinguished obesity researcher Claude Bouchard and his colleagues demonstrates this point very neatly. They took two groups of identical male twins and exposed both members of the pair to a regime of weight gain or weight loss. Some twin pairs were overfed and were put into positive energy balance for a number of weeks. Other pairs were put into negative energy balance by increasing exercise levels while restricting their food intake. The experiments were very well controlled. Not surprisingly all the twins in the first group gained weight and all those in the second group lost weight. But what was striking was that there were enormous differences in how much weight the members of the pairs gained or lost. For example, over 100 days of overfeeding a pair of twins, one twin gained 12 kg, while his sibling only gained 4 kg. Similar variation in weight loss was observed between twins. Clearly, even identical twins, with the same genes, had very different ways of handling a challenge to their metabolism.

Modern medicine does not find such observations very easy to deal with. Doctors, like so many of us, have been seduced by a simple working model—how well you control your weight depends simply on your genes and your behaviour—what you eat, what you choose to do. But clearly it is not as simple as that. If the identical twins studied by Bouchard, who had identical genetic make-up and were made to live in the same way for some weeks, showed such enormous variation in weight control, how can we explain it and what does it mean for the rest of us?

Mr and Mrs Average

Medicine too often ignores such individual variation and focuses on the average. Medical textbooks describe typical cases of disease rather than explaining the full range of ways in which the disease might manifest itself. And medicine tends to assume that we are either sick or we are healthy, with no in-between states. The emphasis of medicine is usually on spotting the definitely abnormal rather than on understanding subtle and not so subtle variations in normality. Typically the latter has been the interest of anthropologists, but there has been surprisingly little interchange between the anthropological and medical communities even though they both study the human condition.

In Bouchard's experiment all of the twins appeared normal yet some of them clearly put on more weight than others when given excess food. So were those rapid weight gainers actually not as healthy as they appeared? Then again, some twins seemed to lose more weight during the negative energy programme than others. Were they in fact unhealthy because they could lose weight too easily? Or might it be the other way around? Perhaps the twins that did not lose very much weight during the exercise programme were the unhealthy ones who might have trouble regulating their body weight later in their lives. Sorting out what is normal starts to become a bit of headache.

In recent years, medicine has taken this concept of the normal versus the abnormal further—we now screen young adults and middle-aged people to determine who already has the early signs of disease—insulin resistance or high blood pressure, for example. But this is really too late in that the person singled out for treatment is already on the pathway to disease; disease is inevitable, and all that can be done is to slow down the journey. Such screening has value but it will not prevent anyone getting the disease, nor indeed will it give us any insights into why we are on a high-risk or low-risk path in the first place. Focusing on the dichotomous approach of early categorization as normal or abnormal does not deal with the key issue, which is understanding why there is variation in the biology of individuals which sets them off on different paths—it seems that there is something in their biology that allows apparently normal people to progress very differently through the risky journey of life.

There are many biological processes that might vary subtly between individuals and affect this journey, yet this variation cannot be considered abnormal even though it may have long-term consequences. The variation could be in appetite control; in food preference; digestion and absorption; in liver or muscle metabolism; in their number of fat cells; how efficiently their hormones work; and so forth. When all is said and done, it is quite difficult to get fat unless we have ready access to food and eat lots of it. It is also quite difficult to become fat if we indulge in intense exercise or intense manual labour on a daily basis. But this does not mean that the reverse is true, and herein lies the problem. Not everyone gets fat despite an indulgent lifestyle. We have seen that there are enormous differences between people. Some of these differences are genetic but the failure of the genetic association studies suggests that most differences are intrinsic in some other way. They are independent of any conscious lifestyle decisions about what to eat and when to exercise. And the complexities pile up: while being obese does lead to a greater risk of heart disease and diabetes, there is not a one-to-one correspondence between being fat and suffering from one of these diseases. Indeed, individual variation confuses the picture at every level. And that leads to the next question: where does this variation come from, if it is not all simply genetic? We address this question in the next chapter.

7

The Child is Father to the Man

Bad time to be born

The Gambia in West Africa is a poor country and most Gambians still depend on subsistence farming for their food supply. It has very consistent weather patterns that lead to dramatic seasonal changes in food supply, so much so that the year can be divided into the 'harvest' season and the 'hungry' season. Pregnant women have had to get used to living on an average of 1,400 calories day through several months of the hungry season but when the harvest comes they can eat about 1,800 calories every day for the next few months. The cycle then starts again. Children, of course, can be born in either season. But what happens to these children as they grow up has been the subject of considerable research. Because The Gambia is so poor, many children die before they are five years old, but there is no difference in the death rates of those born in either of the two very different seasons. Indeed nothing looks very different in terms of mortality until the children reach the age of about 20, when something surprising seems to happen. Those who had been born in the hungry season start to look more fragile, and they become more likely to die of various illnesses than those who had been born in the harvest season. And over time the difference between these two groups of people gets larger and larger—so much so that the average life expectancy of those born in the hungry season is about 15 years shorter than that of those born in the harvest season.

This is an enormous difference. What can be going on? The only explanation must be that something about the conditions at the time they were born or during their early life as a fetus has made them vulnerable—vulnerable in a way that does not affect them obviously in childhood but starts making an enormous difference, literally the difference between life and death, as they reach adulthood. The latency of the effect is revealing. Something in the underlying biology of these babies is influencing the way they will go through life. Something in their biology is being set for life by their mother's nutrition before they are born.

This difference in life expectancy in The Gambia is not the only example we have that suggests a remarkable link between our life before we are born and our journey through life. We have already described the Dutch winter famine of 1944–5 when the Nazis reduced the rations available to the people of the western Netherlands from about 2,000 to about 700 calories per day. The women who were pregnant during the famine gave birth to babies whose birth size was not greatly affected (except for those who were in late pregnancy when the famine started) but those children have grown up to be more at risk of diabetes and cardiovascular disease. The same thing is true of children born at the time of the horrific famine in China in 1958–61, during the so-called Great Leap Forward, when Mao Zedong imposed incredibly destructive policies on the Chinese economy. They too grew up to have a higher risk of diabetes.

These experiments of history and nature are both disturbing and instructive. They are examples of how extreme conditions at the start of life have echoes for the whole of our lives. But this is also true of much less extreme situations. After all, every pregnancy is different—mothers vary in what they eat, how stressed they get, how much exercise they do—and they differ during pregnancy and before. Do these variations in normal pregnancies have long-term consequences for the next generation as well, and if so why?

Paths of destiny

Over the past two decades, a large amount of research has led us to realize that an individual's biological destiny is indeed heavily influenced by what happens to them as an embryo, as a fetus, and as an infant, even in the most unremarkable of pregnancies or infancies. Before we explain that evidence and its implications, it is worth asking why an emphasis on early life should turn out to be so important in the pathway to chronic disease. The simplest answer is a chain of cause and effect: the events in early life change our biology in such a way as to make us respond differently to what we confront later in life.

It is like building a house. If the foundations are not properly laid, no matter what is done after that, problems will emerge sooner or later. A subtle defect in the composition of the concrete used in the foundations may not matter at the beginning but in time it will start to crumble and if there is an earthquake the consequences will be much worse. This is the concept of 'path dependency'—little things at the beginning can have much greater consequences later, in the context of some other event. The analysis of aeroplane crashes and other tragedies shows how disastrously the consequences of path dependency can play out. The space shuttle Challenger was destroyed as a consequence of a very small defect in an O-ring which led to a series of failures on take-off; an event which diminished the thrill of the space age.

So, if path dependency matters in our biology, and if the risk of disease is affected by subtle events that happen early in our lives, our passage through life could be very different if we were able to identify those early changes and the factors causing them. And the evidence for this is accumulating. Indeed, we now know that many of the processes which influence whether or not we are likely to succumb to chronic disease are not only influenced by events in early life but actually start during early life. For example, the number of muscle cells in the heart is definitively set during fetal life. We are all born with our full complement of beating heart muscle cells and these must function for (hopefully) at least two billion heartbeats during our lives. They cannot stop contracting, relaxing, and then contracting again, whether we are reading, exercising intensely, or asleep.

In the same way, the number of filtering units in our kidneys is established before we are born. These will continue to filter our blood every day, removing excess fluid, toxins, and metabolic by-products, and excreting them in the urine. The filtering task is enormous—they do not just secrete urine; they have to filter many litres of blood and in doing so extract much fluid out of our bodies, and then to reabsorb most of that fluid again, because we only pass about 1–2 litres of urine each day. These kidney units, called nephrons, are tremendously active units—they receive about a quarter of the blood pumped by the heart every minute throughout our lives. But as we get older they slowly fail. In most people this is not a problem because we start life with spare capacity, but in some susceptible individuals the rate of decline may be too fast or, more importantly, they started out with a smaller number of filtering units as babies. Either way this deficiency in functioning nephrons is more likely to trigger a rise in blood pressure, because the only way to filter fluid with a smaller number of units is to force blood into them at higher pressure—and this will then have longer-term consequences. If the number of effective units falls too much then only dialysis or a kidney transplant can save us.

Even the number of cells which store white fat (technically called adipocytes) in our bodies is set during early life. Many fat cells are made before we are born and their number is essentially fixed by the time that we are adolescents. Of course they can expand or shrink, depending on how much fat is contained within them, but their number is relatively constant.

The number of brain cells, the number of muscle cells, the number of cells in the pancreas that make insulin . . . they all follow a very similar pattern. Recent research shows that there are stem cells in fat and muscle and in the brain that may allow some new cells to be made under particular conditions but, relative to the total number of cells we need, these are very small effects. Indeed one of the biggest challenges in medical research is to see whether we can find a way to activate these stem cells or to create more of them to help repair organs when they become damaged or aged. Stem cell injections are another possibility and we already use such treatment in cancer whereby blood stem cells from the bone marrow are transplanted into people whose own stem cells have been destroyed by chemotherapy and radiotherapy. There is also experimental work to inject stems cells into damaged hearts to try to repair the dead muscle following a heart attack—it looks promising, but it is not routine care as yet. These techniques offer hope that we may be able to assist the function of bodies at times when their destiny, as set in early life, is beginning to look bleak.

Our hidden lives

The hardest problems to deal with in life are those that we can't see. If you are out for a country walk and you suddenly feel a sharp pain in your arm, you may look down and see a wasp on your arm. This is annoying, but at least you have a clear idea of the nature of the problem. You can decide how to deal with it over the next few days. Does it need an anti-inflammatory cream? Is it getting more swollen and painful? Perhaps you are allergic to wasp stings or maybe the site of the sting is becoming infected. You monitor the situation. Pain in the arm which is not associated with any obvious injury is more worrying. If it persists you will need to seek medical help and this may lead to a long series of investigations. It may be associated with a heart problem; it may be the early sign of a neurological condition; it might be due to a bone tumour . . . or it may just be a sprain, or be inexplicable, and will disappear in a week or so.

So it is with life before birth. It is often said that being born is the second most dangerous time in our lives. Certainly the statistics bear this out because, in the absence of modern medical care, the risk of dying from lack of oxygen or other problems around the time of birth is over 10 per cent. Such deaths can still occur even with the most advanced medical care, but their prevention has been the focus of modern obstetrics and paediatrics, and for those of us in the West it has been a remarkable success story. Fewer than five babies in every 1,000 live births will die in a developed country, and most of those have major medical problems or are born extremely prematurely. Much of that success has come about because we have developed ways of observing the fetus, assessing its health, and then keeping an eye on how it is coping with the dramatic events of being born. And so we can deal with the complications that may occur in the birth process—if necessary, we can perform an emergency Caesarean section, or resuscitate the baby if it is not breathing adequately after birth. One of the most dramatic advances in all of medicine has been the ability to keep premature babies alive. Forty years ago it was rare for any baby born at less that 34 weeks of gestation to survive; now it is routine for babies as young as 26 weeks to survive, and some do so from as early as 22 weeks' gestation (although many of these cases will have less than ideal outcomes).

We can evaluate the health of the fetus remotely using ultrasound or by measuring some critical aspects of fetal life, such as heart rate, via electrodes placed on the mother's abdomen or simply by listening with a stethoscope. We can measure fetal movements. We can use hormone measurements in the mother's blood to ascertain the health of the placenta. If we need to, we can even use a fine needle to draw amniotic fluid from the sac that surrounds the fetus or even fetal blood from the umbilical cord to measure the baby's nutrient, growth factor, and hormone levels. All these methods give us a very good idea of how well the fetus is coping, in much the same way as a paramedic might take measurements of a person at the site of an accident. In the absence of such monitoring, problems can creep up unnoticed and become life-threatening in a very short period of time.

But these are the successes of Western medicine. In much of the world this is not routine practice—sadly, about half a million women die in childbirth or from conditions related to pregnancy every year, and throughout the world a baby under a year old dies from such problems about every 4 seconds; about eight million per year. Less than half the mothers and babies in the world are attended at birth by a trained midwife, and many more than half of all babies at birth do not have the most basic of health assessments made—they are not even weighed.

Birth is the culmination of many months of growth and development within the womb. There is no shortage of challenges or problems which can occur during that time. The fetus appears able to cope with many of these unaided, and in fact it is so good at doing this that we may never know that it has faced any problems at all. But the more we look, the more we find that there are subtle echoes of these experiences that have a cost in terms of later health.

There has been a dramatic change in our understanding of fetal development over about the past 50 years and this has led to a major re-evaluation of the answer to that most fundamental of questions—what makes us what we are? The study of development has emerged as perhaps the most exciting part of modern biology—be it in understanding how one fertilized egg can become the complex being that we are, or the subtleties of how seemingly small differences in developmental experiences can have lifelong effects in making us all different.

Learning in the dark

For most of human history our development before birth remained a complete mystery. The ancient anatomists, such as Galen, dissected the bodies of pregnant women—many of these were condemned criminals and most, but probably not all, were dead at the time—and were able to describe some of the key features of the anatomy of the developing fetus, its placenta, and the environment in which it lived. But we can only learn so much from anatomy. In the absence of anaesthesia or sterile surgical techniques, it was not possible to study developmental function to follow how the fetus grew along its own characteristic path and the adjustments which it made to its structure and function along the way. Knowledge of such adjustments had to wait until the invention of ultrasound and techniques for monitoring fetal growth and development in pregnant animals.

The new knowledge gained by such advances led us to radically revise our ideas about fetal life. Because it was known that the fetus could not survive outside the womb, at least until very late in gestation, it was believed that it must be entirely dependent on its mother, not only for survival but also for the regulation and control of all aspects of its growth and development.

We can see why this idea was so widely believed. All pregnant women detect the movements of their fetuses and can describe the many ways in which the baby seems to respond to what is happening to them—for example, a sudden loud noise such as a passing train may startle the fetus just as much as the mother. The fetus is particularly active after the mother has had a meal, as if it seems to have taken on board more fuel and is now doing some aerobics. In folklore there were many explanations of what are called 'maternal impressions'. For example, if a woman were frightened by a bull in pregnancy, her child was expected to manifest some bovine characteristics. There is absolutely no truth in such stories, but we can see how they might have arisen in an attempt to understand how problems—for example, Siamese twins, or babies born with a cleft palate or a strawberry birth mark—had occurred during the secret life in the womb. This rudimentary folk knowledge gave us very little insight into the way in which the fetus is able to control its own life and influence its destiny.

But fetal life is in fact very different from this. We have now gained enormous insights into all sorts of subtle 'decisions' which control our lives within the womb and influence our destiny after we are born. They are highly sensitive and effective and start very early in gestation, actually when we are still a tiny embryo. The fetus does not merely sit around or doze peacefully during the long months before birth, as if it were waiting for its real life to begin—far from it. It is continuously detecting signals about the world outside, transmitted through the medium of its mother and the placenta, and adjusting the course of its development accordingly. It measures the level of the nutrients which are supplied from the mother across its placenta and responds to the composition and balance of those nutrients. It monitors hormones produced by the mother, sometimes modified by the placenta, and then passed on to it. To a lesser extent, it detects gravity, light and dark, and sound levels. Certainly, if the mother becomes ill with an infection or develops a complication of pregnancy, such as high blood pressure or pre-eclampsia, the fetus will pick up signs of this problem. All this information is used to help the developing baby to adjust to the world in which he or she will live after birth. These signals coming from the mother may be very valuable to the survival of the baby as it grows and develops after it is born. The 'decisions' made by the fetus in adjusting its development are not, of course, conscious, but are intrinsic aspects of our biology—just as the pancreas 'knows' to secrete more insulin when we have high blood sugar levels.

As we develop, these sensing and control mechanisms get more sophisticated. They affect just about every organ of the fetal body in some way or another. We noted the number of urine filtering units in the kidney, and the number of muscle cells in the heart, but they also regulate the density of the bones, the types of fibres in the major muscles of the body, the way in which the pancreas and the liver work to control metabolism, and even how the fetal brain and its later reproductive function will develop. It would appear that the fetus is using its time in the womb to educate itself about what its future life will be like. And the mother is doing her best to teach her fetus about the world in which she lives, on the assumption that this will be the world in which her baby will live too.

When we think of it in these terms, it is obvious that the developmental period of each human being has the potential to confer an enormous advantage on that person later on. Think of the different lives and experiences between an Inuit in Greenland and a Masai in Kenya, or even between someone who lives in a poor village in Uttar Pradesh and someone from the wealthy area of Malabar Hill in Mumbai—these differences could not be more stark. Being prepared for the way of life in these very different conditions will be an enormous advantage.

Be prepared

The better a growing baby is prepared to live in these different environments the better he or she will fare in later life. Being prepared is dependent on making use of the fact that our early development is to some extent plastic. Certain components of our development are, of course, fixed—we have four limbs and 20 digits, our heart is on the left, our thyroid gland makes thyroid hormones rather than adrenaline, and so on. But at a more subtle level there is plasticity in our development, such that subtle environmental changes in fetal and infant life influence many aspects of it. We may end up with finger lengths that are different, we may be taller or shorter, and we will have considerable variation in the number of heart and brain cells and in the sensitivity of the multiple control systems that operate our bodies.

But there is a cost. Because the fetus is sensitive to its environment, there are, unfortunately, circumstances in which the environment provided by the mother is damaging to its development. For example, if she takes the drug thalidomide between 20 and 40 days of pregnancy, the placenta turns that drug into a toxin that affects fetal limb development. That the placenta could turn drugs into poisons was, sadly, not known at the time that thalidomide was developed. Alternatively, sometimes infectious agents get across the placental barrier and damage the fetus; rubella (German measles) is a well-known example, but there are others, such as the bacterium listeria found in some unpasteurized cheeses, or the bacterium that causes syphilis. These agents interfere with the fundamental fetal developmental programme and cause significant disruption of both structure and function—with serious lifelong consequences.

Thankfully these cases of developmental disruption are relatively rare, and they are not our focus. What concerns us here is the range of environmental influences that can alter the pattern of essentially normal development. These are generally more subtle influences and reflect the common range of experiences that a mother might have—from what she eats to her general health or the degree of stress she experiences. Even without dangerous situations such as famine and starvation, sometimes the mother and placenta fail to deliver enough food, or the right balance of nutrients, to the fetus. Then the fetus has to make a decision—how should it allocate its scarce resources? Sometimes it 'decides' to reduce its body growth while maintaining energy supplies to its rapidly growing brain and heart. The result may be a fetus of reduced birth weight. Sometimes it decides to maintain the growth of its liver and to lay down more fat and less muscle. The result is a baby with a different body composition but probably no reduction in birth weight.

The fetal supply line of food is complicated—it is influenced by what the mother eats and her digestion, her reserves in the form of her body composition, her health, and her energy balance.

The nutrients leave her bloodstream and enter the placenta, which consumes some for its own needs and passes the rest on to the fetal bloodstream. The placenta's metabolism is important for exchanging some vital nutrients such as essential amino acids with the fetus. Placental malfunction is common in pre-eclampsia, and that is why fetal growth retardation is often associated with this condition. But every fetus is dependent on its placenta, and the hormonal and metabolic dialogue between the two, about supply and demand, affects fetal development in ways that can have long-term consequences.

Maternal stress can affect the fetus because when stress hormone levels are high, they can overwhelm the normal mechanisms that limit their passage across the placenta. The levels of the stress hormone cortisol (which is made by the adrenal glands) are normally tightly regulated, and the fetus generally has very low levels of cortisol until late in gestation, when its production by the fetus starts to increase in the run-up to birth. Babies born prematurely do not have high enough cortisol levels and this makes their survival risky, because the hormone prepares the fetus for birth by maturing organs such as the lungs. This discovery in the 1970s was arguably the most important in neonatal medicine. Sir Graham (Mont) Liggins in Auckland found that an artificial form of cortisol could bypass the placental barrier and, when given to a woman in premature labour, would accelerate her baby's lung maturation. Overnight, the survival of many premature babies became possible. Much modern neonatal medicine is based on refinements of this discovery, which has saved hundreds of thousands of lives.

The causes of premature labour are poorly understood. One common cause is infection which can ascend from the vagina and pass through the protective membranes around the fetus, releasing chemicals that initiate labour. The fetus in this situation is better out of the dangerous infected environment, and so 'makes' the choice to be born prematurely, to have at least some chance of survival. In evolutionary terms this trade-off could only have worked for a small degree of prematurity—perhaps only after a pregnancy duration of 37 weeks or so.

Other causes of premature delivery reflect the conditions of the mother early in pregnancy. We now know that mothers who are inadequately nourished at this time are more likely to give birth a few weeks prematurely. Indeed, across the developing world pregnancy lengths are often one to two weeks shorter than in the developed world. As we shall see, this brings with it a cost. We also know that mothers who experience severe stress, such as surviving an earthquake, have a shorter length of pregnancy. But the surprising finding is that it is those women who suffered the traumatic experience in early pregnancy who have the earlier births. The fact that gestational length is influenced by events in early pregnancy suggests that the tempo of fetal development is set in early embryonic life.

Some simple experiments make this point very clear. Farm animals such as sheep often give birth to twins, or even triplets, and every sheep farmer knows that these will be smaller than singleton animals. For many years it was thought that this was because nutrient supply, and even physical space, was less for each fetal lamb if a twin or triplet than if they had the uterus, the mother, and the placenta to themselves. But then a researcher, Frank Bloomfield in Auckland, decided to ask a very simple question. At what rate would a twin sheep fetus grow if its other twin was removed or died in early gestation? Would it grow at the same rate as a singleton fetus, as it now had no competition, or would it grow at the rate of a twin, as it was actually conceived? The answer was clear and surprising—the surviving twin still grew at the rate of a twin, as if it did not know that it had its mother's resources all to itself. Clearly, aspects of fetal growth and development are established very early in pregnancy.

So embryos and fetuses use information derived from the mother to predict what kind of nutrition they will receive or how much stress they will be exposed to after birth. They then use the fact that development is plastic or flexible to shift the set points in their metabolic and stress control systems so as to be better placed to thrive in the world into which they predict they will be born. They will not get it right all the time and, as we will see, this has consequences. But as they *do* get it right more often than not, evolution has preserved these plastic mechanisms. Practically all multicellular organisms have some form of a developmental phase, and in every type of animal studied so far (and indeed in many plants too), developmental plasticity is used to establish a strategy to optimize fitness from early on in the life-course.

Evolving to breed

What is the meaning of such a life-course strategy? Quite simply, that we can't do everything in our lives to perfection and so it is necessary to make choices to concentrate more on certain aspects and less on others. In other words we have to make trade-offs, and the most powerful ones which all complex organisms make are between investing resources for reproduction as opposed to investing them in the repair and maintenance necessary for longevity.

We need to examine this idea. Does it mean that a developing organism should invest all available resources in its future reproduction? And what do we mean by reproduction? The answer is not as simple as investing in sperm and egg machines. Successful reproduction is about much more. We must survive to and through sexual maturation; we must attract an appropriate mate; and we must survive long enough for our offspring themselves to be independent and reproduce—otherwise our genes will not persist, and, in evolutionary terms, that is what life is about.

Accordingly, the balance of survival and reproductive strategies varies enormously between animal species. But every one has a strategy which balances successful reproductive potential against the contingencies of the ecological niche in which the species finds itself. Critical phases of our evolution occurred in Africa five to six million years ago, when we diverged in our ancestry from the other great apes, and then perhaps 160,000 years ago when modern Homo sapiens first emerged. Of our last 160,000 years—which equates to perhaps 8,000 generations—most was in the so-called Palaeolithic period. Agriculture and settlement only appeared 10,000 years ago (some 500 generations) in the Middle East, and more recently else-where. This was the Neolithic period. But in contrast to these long periods of our evolutionary past which shaped our biology, many of the issues we are concerned with in this book relate to the last 100 years—the last four generations or fewer.

While we can only speculate about the patterns of reproductive behaviour in our Palaeolithic ancestors, anthropologists have enough clues to arrive at a consensus. First, females would have mated soon after puberty. Those women in better nutritional condition would be more likely to survive; those who were of larger build would be less likely to have an obstructed labour. Males probably competed for females either by social dominance, for example by being head of the clan, or possibly by sheer physical dominance over other males. In many hunter-gatherer societies physical prowess determines social dominance, so we can surmise that strong and large males had a greater role in creating the human gene pool in the Palaeolithic period.

In evolutionary terms, survival up until the time of reproduction is critical for both males and females. It is pointless to come to within a few months of achieving puberty and then succumb to an infection or an injury. So we have evolved with a strategy such that our grow-ing bodies also invest considerable resources in repair and defence mechanisms, whether they are the processes of immunity by which we fight off invading bacteria and viruses or the processes by which damage to our DNA is repaired following the accidents which happen to it during cell division. But doing this effectively up to the time of reproduction leads to a trade-off against having as much capacity to do so later in life.

The balance between how much resource to invest in growth and reproductive function and how much to invest in repair and restoration later in life is thus a classic life history trade-off. The important point is that the equilibrium involved in this trade-off can be shifted if environmental circumstances change. This has been extremely well demonstrated in many animal species. For example, many amphibians, such as the spadefoot toad, will trade off between growth and the timing of metamorphosis from a tadpole into an adult if they are challenged with harsh environmental conditions. Suppose that the pond in which the tadpoles are living in the Arizonan desert begins to dry up. Clearly it is time to leave the pond and make the best of it on land. So the metamorphosis of the tadpoles is accelerated, and they become young toads in order to leave the pond. As a result, they become reproductively competent at a younger age even though they are smaller as adult toads. This is a risky strategy because smaller animals are more likely to be picked off by predators such as snakes or birds but it is a gamble that has to be taken if there is to be any chance of reproduction. To stay as a tadpole when the pond has dried up is certain death. It is no good waiting to grow to a certain size before reproducing if waiting will be fatal.

There is a range of threatening situations in life which can evoke a similar strategy. For example, in guppies (the little fish often seen in aquaria) that live in the wild, the presence of high numbers of predators induces early puberty in the male guppy. These guppies reproduce early and abundantly, even though they are small, and are then likely to die earlier.

And it looks as if humans do the same thing as well. Puberty can be best studied in females, as the age at the first period, or menarche, is a reliable and clear measure of sexual maturation. A study by a number of anthropologists of modern hunter-gatherer communities has looked at the age at menarche and related it to the likelihood of mortality at a young age in those communities. These hunter-gatherer societies are small groups of people in the Amazon, New Guinea, and Central Africa who have lives somewhat similar to those who lived before modern technologies and colonization. Of course their lives are not exactly as they were 2,000 years ago, and often they have been displaced from their ancestral homes, but this study does give us some insights into Neolithic society and biology. It turns out that in those societies, where there is a high risk of juvenile death, the age at menarche can be as much as six years earlier than in those societies where the juvenile mortality is low.

But if the decision is made to reproduce early, and this must be at the cost of the body's growth and repair systems, what might be the longer-term consequences? For the spadefoot toads it is a greater risk of death by predation. But what about humans? As we discussed in the last chapter, while our expected lifespan—except in the least developed world—is now in the order of seven to nine decades, in our evolutionary past most individuals probably lived no more than three to five decades. And it was through those 8,000 generations of the Palaeolithic that our biology evolved. It was 'designed' to make trade-off decisions about surviving to reproduce and to support our children until they reached the age of independence. We estimate that this meant that we evolved to live for about 35 to 50 years.

How did we arrive at this figure? The best evidence comes from the study of female reproduction. By the age of 35, even well-nourished healthy women in the most developed societies show a decline in fertility—the chances of getting pregnant even with unprotected intercourse at the optimal time in the menstrual cycle starts to decline. In most women, by the age of about 50 the ovaries have ceased to release eggs altogether and menopause occurs. In hunter-gatherer societies menopause tends to be closer to 40 years. Presumably, in evolutionary terms women by that age are likely to have had sufficient children—even though up to half of them may have died—to sustain the lineage. Following the cessation of reproduction, women in early human societies would have had to survive for at least another decade to support their youngest child to reproductive maturity. If the youngest child was a girl, there may have been a further evolutionary advantage in the woman surviving long enough for her grandchildren to reach maturity. This suggests an evolved average life expectancy of around 50 years of age. Males, on average, enter puberty later than females and have shorter lives, but examination of modern athletes suggests that males in early human societies would most likely have had peak physical performance in their thirties. Probably many of them did not live much beyond this age.

Clearly most of our Palaeolithic ancestors did not die of old age, although some of them did live well into their later years. We imagine that senile dementia, Alzheimer's disease, or even the fractured hips of the elderly, regrettably so common today, were a rarity then. Most deaths, presumably, occurred from infection and injury through accident or violence. Death in childbirth was also common—perhaps affecting 10 per cent of all women. In any event we did not evolve to live even the three score years and ten quoted in the Bible. This may explain why the common chronic non-communicable diseases which we associate with ageing today—cancer, cardiovascular disease, stroke, dementia, and osteoporosis—are so difficult to treat. All of these diseases have a pathological component which results from an inability to repair damaged biology.

So we can see the result of the trade-off: in order to achieve reproductive success earlier in our lives, we evolved the biological strategy of trading off the repair and restoration processes which we will need in middle and old age. The gamble paid off in terms of human evolution and colonization of the world, but every older person now has to pay the price.

Royals and commoners

The data on the hunter-gatherers we described earlier in this chapter give compelling evidence that trade-offs between reproduction and ageing actually exist in humans. But can we find other evidence? One way of looking at the problem is to see if there are historical records which allow us to relate reproductive success to lifespan in Western populations over a long period of time. Do such records exist? Tom Kirkwood and his colleagues in Newcastle focused on the records that have been kept for the English aristocracy. In view of the importance of succession in the British royal family, it is clear that even several hundred years ago such records would be accurate as they would not have been for other members of society. In addition, we imagine that at any time in history the royal family has had access to the best available nutrition and so, if the biological trade-offs operate in this family, we would expect them to be less obscured by other complicating factors. Kirkwood and colleagues found that such trade-offs do indeed exist.

In the English aristocracy, life expectancy was greater for women who had fewer children and lower for those who had more. It was also high for those who had their first child at a later age. So having more children (and starting to have them earlier) is associated with a shorter life. Of course, these data relate to only one family, but the trends are in the direction predicted by evolutionary biology.

Nobody would claim that the lives of the English aristocracy are representative of human existence across the globe, or even in the UK itself, especially over a historical timescale. More recent attempts to address this problem have come from the work of the evolutionary psychologist Daniel Nettle, who also works in Newcastle. Nettle used data from the Millennium Cohort Study which comprised 8,660 families in the UK, in which social and other factors were measured across the population, from the most deprived to the most affluent neighbourhoods. He was able to show that, compared with affluent families, in more deprived neighbourhoods the age at first birth is younger, birth weights are lower, and breastfeeding duration is shorter. He also found some evidence that reproductive rates are higher—giving larger family size. He interprets his work as a modern-day human equivalent of the trade-offs we discussed for animals. But here the challenge is poverty and poorer social circumstances leading to earlier, and perhaps more frequent, reproduction.

The broader social consequences of such processes, if they can be shown to operate more widely across society, are extremely important. The children of younger mothers, especially in low-income settings, are less likely to do as well at school or to have the same level of lifetime earnings as those of the older mothers of affluent families. They are also less likely to have their father resident in the home or even to have as much contact with their maternal grandmothers. These effects have the potential to be extremely costly for society in humanitarian as well as financial terms, and the fact that they still operate in the UK today is very worrying. Poverty and social deprivation beget poverty and social deprivation, and breaking this cycle is extremely difficult, as every recent UK government has experienced. To a degree every recent UK government has also failed to meet this challenge because the gap between the rich and the poor, in terms of access to education, healthcare, and financial stability, is greater today than it was when the welfare state was founded just after the Second World War.

Dan Nettle's provocative study does not give us any insight into the underlying unconscious mechanisms which are operating, and in some respects this makes it quite difficult to predict which individuals or population groups will be at particular risk. And the data are subject to alternative interpretations. This is the difficulty of such research—studying humans is much more complex than studying experimental animals where the conditions can be controlled. But on the other hand, humans are animals too, and if we can obtain strong data in other species and suggestive data in humans then we can be moderately certain that the conclusions reached apply to us too.

If life history trade-offs are operative in modern Western societies, then we would expect to see that girls who had a poorer start to life, and thus whose biology was tuned by prediction of a shorter lifespan, would be younger at menarche. Furthermore, as there is no reproductive value in reaching menarche early unless one is in a good enough physical condition to support an early pregnancy, we believe that the earliest age at menarche would be seen in those who were born smallest—that is, had a poor start to life—and then developed relative fatness in childhood. We developed this concept from a series of studies made in rats and from trying to make sense of a rather disparate group of studies in humans. But more recently this concept was validated in a study in Western Australia led by John Newnham. Deborah Sloboda and her fellow researchers divided a group of almost 1,000 girls into subgroups based on their weight at birth and their weight at seven years of age. They found that the earliest menarche occurred in the girls of lowest birth weight and greatest weight at seven years. The latest menarche was in the opposite subgroup—girls of highest birth weight and lowest childhood weight gain. The difference in the timing of menarche between these two extremes was more than a year, which is a very substantial effect in evolutionary—and in modern social—terms when looking across a population.

Imagine a class of 11-year-olds just starting secondary school, where perhaps a third of the girls have already started to have regular monthly periods, but another third show no signs of menarche at all. Their relationships and reactions to the boys in the class will be substantially different, as of course might be the consequences. Needless to say, many studies have confirmed that girls who have menarche earlier are engaged in sexual activities at a younger age. Other studies from Europe have shown that both boys and girls who have earlier puberty are at greater risk of behavioural and mental health problems: in girls, eating disorders, and in boys, even suicide. These are serious matters, and while they are not all related to puberty and sexual activity, the fact that a high proportion of them are raises concerns.

The continuum

There is something else which is reflected in the findings from Western Australia: size at birth is not everything—just being bigger is not necessarily better than being smaller. As we will soon discuss in detail, many population studies around the world have shown that the risk of cardiovascular disease and diabetes is greater in people who were smaller than average at birth. Equally the risk of some forms of cancer in later life is greater in those who were larger babies at birth. And, as we will discuss in the next chapters, babies who are very big are likely to have mothers who had diabetes in pregnancy, and this in turn puts them at greater risk of developing diabetes themselves. Developmental processes act as a continuum. Even if we take a simple measure of development such as weight at birth, we can see that there is a spectrum of consequences which follow. The Western Australia study shows that this is so even across the normal birth weight range—a point of major importance.

Add to this idea the fact that life itself is a continuum, and we can see that decisions and strategies established at one point in life, say in prenatal development, can have consequences a long way down the track. The types of chronic disease which develop, their nature, and the time in life at which they occur vary enormously between individuals. We all travel on different trajectories through our lives and what happens to us at one point in time, from our early development onwards, will have consequences much later.

This idea does not just apply to developed, high-income societies. One of the best examples, which demonstrates this concept dramatically, is the study from The Gambia which we discussed at the start of this chapter. The seasonal effect on mortality does not become evident until after the time of reproduction, when the trade-off produced by a poor start to life—developing and being born in the hungry season—leads to greater mortality later.

So what happens to us at the very start of life can impact on our destiny through the rest of our lives. These effects are not matters of extremes—of disruptions to our developmental programme such as those induced by measles infection or poisons during pregnancy. Rather, they are the echo of our evolutionary past, and utilize the processes of developmental plasticity, whereby every developing organism tries to take information from its developmental environment to predict its future, and to prepare itself accordingly. Now we need to explore what happens when a fetus predicts a good environment and what happens when it predicts a bad environment—for within this may lie the clues to the missing factor that explains why some of us get fat more easily, and some of us suffer from diabetes and cardiovascular disease, while others do not.

8

Trouble Ahead

Simple minds

For too long, the role of development in biomedical science and clinical medicine has been played down. For many years scientific research on development has been seen as the poor cousin, or perhaps we should say the poor son or daughter, of studies of the biology of adult organisms, including humans. One of the authors remembers overhearing a remark made by a very eminent professor during a break in a scientific meeting. It coincided with the time at which the author was deciding to switch to research in developmental physiology himself. His illustrious senior must have been discussing with a colleague a paper or a research funding application which they had both been sent to review. 'Oh well, of course you don't have to be very clever to work on development,' he said. 'After all, it's much simpler than adult biology.' The other author was told by his distinguished Professor of Medicine when he decided to be a paediatrician that he was

136

throwing his career as a medical scientist away—'Nothing fundamental or important ever comes out of paediatrics,' he said.

Such disparaging remarks were familiar to those of us who have built careers in developmental physiology and medicine—the dominant idea was that development was merely a process of assembly of simple components, uninteresting in themselves, which merited the attention of the greatest intellects in science only when they were put together to form the adult organism. Bizarre as it might seem now, babies were seen as simpler versions of adults—and so the medical problems of children were regarded as simpler than the medical problems of adults.

To those biomedical scientists who insisted on looking at development through the wrong end of the telescope, it has come as an enormous surprise that there are highly complex processes operating during this period of our lives, some of which are unique to development itself. They were shocked to discover that the fetus has a good deal of control over its destiny and even the very processes of its development, while it is undergoing them. Development is not like a car being assembled on a production line from bins of identical parts, which has no role or function until the assembly is complete and it can be driven.

Even more surprising to those solely focused on the adult has been the revelation that many developmental processes play a critical role in evolution. Not only have they evolved to fulfil specific fitness functions, but they also play a major part in influencing Darwinian fitness itself. This realization has caused a major revolution in evolutionary thought.

We are relieved that such blinkered views are now very rare, and developmental biology is recognized as one of the most exciting areas of modern science.

We have now come to the point in our story where we need to be specific about the ways in which early human development contributes to the increased risk of obesity and the chronic diseases.

In view of what we have just said, it should not be a surprise that this developmental aspect too was ignored for so long. Is it still being ignored? Let's look at the evidence and then return to that question.

A poor start

There are really two lines of evidence which have demonstrated beyond a shadow of a doubt that early life processes play a major role in influencing obesity and non-communicable disease risk. Let us consider studies of human populations first. The first studies were made in England in the 1930s, and suggested that children who had poor early development had a high later risk of heart attack. The significance of these observations seems to have been overlooked or forgotten. Then in the 1980s three groups, two in England and one in Sweden, led by Michael Wadsworth, David Barker, and Gerhard Gennser, respectively, reported at about the same time that children who were born at the small end of the normal range had a higher risk of developing high blood pressure as adults.

While the other two groups made the observation and passed on, David Barker, a Southampton physician and epidemiologist, was not content with just making the observation only once. He conducted a series of compelling observations in many communities and started on an important mission: trying to persuade the medical community that the problems their patients faced started before they were born. His observations were dismissed as flukes, as confused by uncontrolled factors, and as scientifically implausible. How could factors operating before we were born influence our risk of disease 50–60 years later? However, gradually more and more population scientists began to confirm Barker's findings. They extended the observations from cardiovascular disease to diabetes and then to insulin resistance in children, an early sign of adult diabetes.

Even after these concepts had been accepted they were still considered to be of relatively minor importance. It was not clear how a pathway to disease could start with low birth weight. And in any case the fraction of infants in any population born small was low, whereas diabetes and heart disease were becoming so common that in some societies up to 50 per cent of the population suffered from them.

These criticisms were based on fundamental misunderstandings which, it seems to us, would have been quickly addressed in any other field. These epidemiological observations were, in time, clarified so that they made no claim for a link between low birth weight itself and later disease—in fact, what they showed was that processes operating *before* birth were linked to later disease risk. Birth weight is a marker of the prenatal environment, made at the earliest time when it is possible to obtain some direct measurements of the developing baby. Even more important is the fact that the observations did not only concern low birth weight babies. The original observations, along with those of many other studies conducted by scientists in many countries, some of which involved over 100,000 subjects, showed that the risk of later disease was graded across the entire range of normal birth weights. For example, in Barker's studies of men and women born before the Second World War, someone who had been a perfectly normal baby weighing 7.5 pounds at birth was at greater risk than someone who had been an 8-pound baby, whose risk in turn was less than that of an 8.5-pound baby.

Rodent prophets

The other line of evidence comes from studies on animals, mostly rats and mice. In such laboratory animals, which breed rapidly and have a lifespan that usually does not exceed two years, it is much easier to study effects of early development on adult health than it is in human populations. It has been shown repeatedly that reducing the level of food consumed by pregnant rats or mice, either in terms of the total amount of food or just in its protein content, produces long-term effects on their offspring. These include high blood pressure, insulin resistance, a tendency to deposit fat, altered behavioural responses to stress, reduced activity, and even reduced ability to learn new tasks. This collection of characteristics is highly reminiscent of some of the problems experienced by humans who have conditions such as metabolic syndrome. There are even effects on reproduction and ageing. The offspring can develop osteoporosis, kidney failure, and die at an earlier age.

Many of the fundamental experiments in this field were conducted in our laboratories in Southampton and in Auckland, and our colleagues there have gone on to study in detail the mechanisms underlying these processes. One very striking observation comes from experiments in which the diets of the pregnant rat or mouse and of her subsequent offspring were manipulated experimentally to be very different—mismatched—so that the levels of nutrition the same animal was exposed to as a fetus and then after weaning were discordant. For example, if the pregnant animals were fed an inadequate diet, in terms of either its amount or its protein content, while their growing offspring were fed a diet rich in calories or fat, these offspring became obese and developed the equivalent of metabolic syndrome rapidly. But the key point—which was quickly realized in these labs by scientists such as Mark Vickers and Graham Burdge— was that these animals developed the unhealthy conditions more quickly and more severely than animals whose mothers had been well-nourished during pregnancy but which were also fed the high-calorie or high-fat diet as they grew up. It was as if the relative undernourishment during development had primed them to get fat, develop insulin resistance, and so forth more quickly when they were confronted with a high-fat or high-calorie diet. The speed and magnitude of the problem depended on the degree of the mismatch between their mother's diet and the diet that they consumed themselves.

These observations have been confirmed many times by other laboratories. But when we see an important biological phenomenon it is important to shift from the observation itself to ask what it means and *why* it happens. Only then can the observation be truly put in context. As we saw, the ultimate answer to *why* questions generally comes from evolutionary biology, and so we should use evolutionary theory to try to explain what is going on.

Our predictive adaptive response theory proposes that aspects of the mother's environment, including her nutritional status, stress levels, and the number of predators and other threatening events which occur during her pregnancy, are transformed into signals which she sends to her developing fetus. These signals in turn affect the development of her fetus in many ways. The effects do not disrupt development, but they tune it in terms of the relative sizes of the growing organs, the numbers of muscle cells in the heart or of filtering units in the kidney, the extent of fat deposition in the body, and even the levels at which some of its physiological control systems will be set, such as appetite and stress responses. All these developmental processes are made in expectation of the fetus living in an environment similar to that of its mother after it is born and as it grows up. She has educated her baby about the world in which she lives, and this information will be of great importance to her child as he or she grows up. This forecasting (or predictive) strategy is present in humans as well as in many other mammals, and even in some amphibians, plants, and insects.

A good example of this strategy at work can be observed in the little Pennsylvania meadow vole. Because it can be born in either spring or autumn, the baby vole needs to know whether it should be born with a thick or a thin coat of fur, to be prepared for either the cold winter or the hot summer that is coming. The vole has to set the type and the density of its hair follicles before it is born. But it cannot use temperature clues directly, because the temperature in the womb and in the nest is very similar throughout the year. It is only after it leaves the nest that its thick or thin coat becomes important for survival. If it does not survive the winter or summer it will not reproduce, so there is an evolutionary advantage to getting this right. So the vole has evolved the ability to predict whether summer or winter is coming while it is still a fetus. It does so by sensing its mother's melatonin levels, which show a different pattern if the days are shortening as winter comes on, or lengthening as summer approaches. This is a fairly safe prediction—hard to get wrong—but it illustrates the simple point that animals make biological decisions early in development which have long-term consequences for their survival, health, and reproductive success.

There are many examples of these predictive processes in insects. Some butterflies develop very different wing colourations depending on the season in which they hatch. The temperature the larva is exposed to changes the biochemical signals that determine wing colouration. The larva picks up the signal about the season and the changes occur during metamorphosis and development of the wing, but the advantage of altered wing colouration only comes later when the butterfly is mature. Leaf colouration is different in different seasons and it is essential to have the right wing colours for camouflage and to hide from predators.

So we proposed that the human fetus was responding to signals for, say, a nutritionally rich or nutritionally poor future environment and set its physiology accordingly. But when a fetus which predicted a nutritionally poor environment was actually faced with a nutritionally rich environment, its physiology would not be correctly tuned and obesity and all the other problems ensued.

This is all very well, but these ideas are based purely on observations—things which happen in nature and for which it is possible to provide a plausible explanation. But how can we be sure that this is the correct or even the best explanation? We need to go back to the lab and conduct further experiments to test the theory. This is precisely what Mark Vickers and his colleagues did in

Auckland. They reasoned that if the development of the newborn rat pup had been influenced by its mother's diet, and that this would affect the likelihood of its becoming obese when it was given a high-fat diet, then it ought to be possible to prevent or reverse this process by sending a counter-signal at an appropriate time. Suppose, for example, that it was possible to trick the newborn pups into believing that they were already obese very soon after they were born. Would this somehow counteract the signals that they had received before birth and prevent them becoming obese later?

Vickers and colleagues tested this idea directly by giving newborn pups injections of the hormone leptin. We saw earlier in the book that this hormone is produced by fat and acts on the areas of the brain which control appetite. So high levels of leptin should indicate to the growing brain of the newborn rat that it is not hungry and in fact is already relatively obese. When Vickers conducted these experiments the effects were dramatic. The leptin injections completely prevented pups whose mothers had been fed a poor diet during pregnancy from becoming obese—even if they were fed high-fat diets. It also prevented them from developing insulin resistance and high blood pressure, and made them more active and less anxious. Leptin had effectively corrected the message which the developing animals had received from their mothers, based on the poor diet which the mothers were fed. They no longer over-ate the high-fat diet and so did not become obese or develop the characteristics equivalent to human metabolic syndrome. It certainly looked as if the predictive adaptive response theory applied well to rats.

Mismatched people

So far, so good, for the theory. Now we had to go back to look for evidence to support this concept of the mismatch pathway in humans. The confirmation came from some work we undertook with Terrence Forrester, who directs one of the world's most famous nutritional research centres, the Tropical Metabolism Research Unit in Kingston, Jamaica. This Unit was set up after the Second World War, when Jamaica was still a British colony. There was an extraordinarily high level of under-nutrition there, as emphasized by the Unit's first director, John Waterlow, one of the founders of the modern science of nutrition, who died only recently.

Jamaica still has a high incidence of severe infant malnutrition, and children are admitted to Forrester's ward in the hospital in a terrible nutritional state every week. Many families live on the edge of poverty and only one thing needs to happen—the father loses his job or leaves the home, the mother has another child, a hurricane strikes, or just that the child gets an infection—and the child's nutritional state collapses. Severely malnourished children may develop one of two syndromes: marasmus or kwashiorkor. Infants with marasmus look terribly emaciated, with their muscles wasted away. Infants with kwashiorkor have swollen bodies with pot bellies distended by fluid accumulation. We have all seen such children in the heart-rending pictures of famines in Africa. Infants with kwashiorkor are more likely to die. But tragically, even though they die of malnutrition, they still have fuel stores left in the muscle and fat in their bodies. It is as if they cannot mobilize their fuel supplies, unlike the marasmic children who seem to cling onto life, getting thinner and thinner, until there is no more fuel left to burn.

But no one really understood why some infants develop marasmus and others get kwashiorkor—there had been many theories but none satisfactorily explained the difference. They seem to come from similar families and to be exposed to similar levels of under-nutrition. Then Forrester thought of looking back at their birth weights. And there an explanation lay, for marasmic children had lower birth weights than those who developed kwashiorkor. It seemed that fetuses who were less well nourished before birth, and therefore grew less and had a lower birth weight, had predicted a poor nutritional environment and had adjusted their physiology to be good at mobilizing their fuel supplies to withstand famine. When famine struck they developed marasmus—becoming terribly thin, but often surviving. In contrast, fetuses who were better nourished and had higher birth weights had not predicted such famine. When it struck they were not so well prepared, developed kwashiorkor, and had a higher chance of dying. For those children, making the right prediction was a matter of life and death.

Would it be possible to get even more direct proof of the predictive adaptive response theory in Jamaica? Vickers' rats had shown different regulation of appetite according to whether they predicted good or bad times, based on their mother's diet. If our prediction idea was right we would expect to see that survivors of kwashiorkor and marasmus in Jamaica had different appetite control. We decided to test this idea.

The ecologist David Raubenheimer is South African by birth. The media have dubbed him the Indiana Jones of nutrition. After some years in Oxford he emigrated to New Zealand. He now spends his life in exotic places studying the control of food intake in animals ranging from locusts to snow leopards, from lizards to lemurs. He worked closely with Steve Simpson—who is now at the University of Sydney, but was for some time curator at Oxford University's Museum of Natural History, where Thomas Huxley had defended Darwin's ideas against the disbelieving Bishop of Oxford. Raubenheimer and Simpson had developed a very precise method of studying appetite control. It worked in creatures ranging from plague locusts to Oxford medical students. So we enlisted Raubenheimer's help to see if the appetite control of Jamaican children differed according to their developmental history.

In Jamaica, Raubenheimer and Forrester carefully measured appetite control in a group of survivors of famine, who had suffered either kwashiorkor or marasmus as young children. These people are now between 25 and 40 years of age. Sure enough, those people who had predicted a bad environment based on their prenatal cues had very different appetite control mechanisms from those of higher birth size, just as with Mark Vickers' rats.

Clear though this seems, our predictive adaptive response idea has met with some criticisms. The main criticism has come from those researchers who said it was unlikely that the fetus would shift its development for such a long-term advantage. They argued that preserving the mother's health would be much more important. The argument disappeared when it became clear from mathematical modelling that the major determinant of reproductive success in humans is survival to puberty, so the adaptive advantages of predicting and surviving the childhood environment are indeed large. Another argument, that any conflict for resources between the mother and the fetus must be resolved in favour of the mother, also disappeared—mothers do not sacrifice fetal growth, or indeed breast milk production, even during times of extreme famine. Even under horrific wartime conditions, in refugee camps and famine conditions, babies can be born of normal size, and breast milk production is protected. And, importantly, fetuses do not have to be small at birth to have made predictions about their future. It seems that the forecasting or prediction process forms part of normal human biology.

Other data had already pointed in this direction. Many studies have been done on the Dutch Hunger Winter, as we saw earlier. The famine lasted for seven months from late 1944 until the Allies liberated the Netherlands in 1945. Throughout this period Dutch nurses and doctors continued to keep careful records on births. Thanks to the dedication of researchers such as Tessa Roseboom, many of these children have now been followed into middle age. It turns out that those who were born to mothers who were pregnant during the famine are much more likely to become obese and diabetic in middle age—the mismatch effect again. But those who were only exposed to famine for the first third of their gestation, because they were conceived late in the war, did not have reduced birth weights. The argument that the fetus is sacrificed for the mother is thus untenable.

However, the most impressive data on these ideas have come from long-term prospective studies of Western populations, conducted in Southampton. These were originally conceived by David Barker's team and are now run by Hazel Inskip and Keith Godfrey. Their originality lies in the fact that they start making measurements of women, their partners, and often their parents too, before the women become pregnant. This is a major undertaking because, of course, not all the women do become pregnant. In one of their studies, 12,500 women were recruited and studied in detail and the 3,150 who became pregnant were then followed up.

The Southampton studies have shown clearly that birth weight is not the most important factor in setting the risk of chronic disease. The thickness of the carotid artery of a child at nine years of age, an early and highly objective marker of risk of cardiovascular disease, was statistically related to low carbohydrate intake by the mother in late pregnancy, and this effect was independent of the child's birth weight. In other words, the fetus can change its biology on the basis of its mother's diet without necessarily changing its body size overall.

Why do we get the forecast wrong?

If this phenomenon is important in the epidemic of diabetes and cardiovascular disease, we need to explain why so many apparently unremarkable pregnancies are associated with getting the forecast wrong. If we are right, many fetuses are mismatched to the world because they predict a poor nutritional environment but are in reality born into a world of plenty, a world they did not really expect.

What a mother eats or how stressed she is need not necessarily be transmitted accurately all the time to her fetus. After all, the fetus is not directly connected to its mother; there is an intermediate organ—the placenta. And so the transduction of signals about the world out there is dampened and can be distorted. It is like trying to see the world with very primitive radar rather than with your own eyes. You will get an impression, but some things will be missed and others may be misleading. But just as radar, even in its most primitive form, was of value to the air forces and navies of the Second World War, so the information that the fetus can glean from its mother can be valuable to it.

There are many ways in which the information can be misleading. One possibility is that the mother is unwell and is consuming nutritional supplies for herself, or she may have high stress hormone levels.

Another possibility is that the placenta is not working well and thus nutrient transfer is diminished even though the mother has ample supplies. These situations can lead to either premature birth or a reduction in fetal growth, which in turn leads to greater risk of obesity and chronic disease. That might add to risk in perhaps 5–10 per cent of the population but, as the incidence of diabetes and cardiovascular disease is much higher than this, there must be more to the problem than just maternal or placental disease.

One of the many things measured in the Southampton Women's Survey was the food intake of women before conception. What is worrying is that many women do not eat a balanced diet to support their pregnancy. Indeed more that 50 per cent of the women of lowest educational achievement had a diet that was unbalanced. Among those with a university degree it was about 3 per cent. These are very revealing data—they tell us that unbalanced nutrition from the fetal perspective is not just a concern in the least developed world; it is an issue in Western societies as well.

Sometimes the mother's behaviour can also affect birth weight. Over the last 30 years in Japan birth weight has been falling, as we discussed in Chapter 5. One reason for this is that more women now smoke; another is that they have drastically reduced the weight they put on during pregnancy, from about 12 kg to about 8 kg. In Japan, until recently obstetricians recommended only a low level of weight gain in pregnancy even in women who are already very thin. Because of the possible long-term health effects on the next generation produced by such a mismatch, and because of the problems of maternal obesity (which we will investigate in the next chapter), major medical authorities and researchers are now revising their recommendations for weight gain during pregnancy. In general, except under conditions of gross maternal obesity, we hope that all women would gain at least 10–12 kg during their pregnancy.

Keeping the baby under control

But there may be more fundamental reasons why nearly all of us now get the forecast wrong to a certain degree. One is that many of us are first-born. Some years ago we theorized that first-born children would be more at risk of becoming obese, because the nutritional and physical environment of the uterus is more constrained in first than in subsequent pregnancies. So first children would be more likely to predict a nutritionally limited world and thus be mismatched in a modern energy-dense world. This was primarily an evolutionary argument but, if we were right, then it could be playing a major role in the current chronic disease epidemic. More of the world's population is now first-born because, as developing societies go through socio-economic transition, family size has fallen. As family size falls the proportion of those who are first-born inevitably rises. In Singapore, for example, the average number of children in a family is now less than 1.5 per family. In Europe, where the number of children has fallen on average well below two per family, more than half the children are first-born. In urban China this has reached almost 100 per cent through the one-child policy and this, if we are right, might have something to do with explaining the rapid increase of diabetes of China.

Recently our idea has been put to the test. In the early 1950s, a doctor in Motherwell in southern Scotland made substantial recommendations about the diet that his women patients should eat during pregnancy. The offspring were studied until they were 30. Keith Godfrey and his team in Southampton analysed how fat these 30-year-olds were from the point of view of whether they were first-born or not. As we predicted, those who were first-born have about 25 per cent more body fat than those who were second or subsequent children. Most recently, data from Cesar Victora's group in Brazil have shown that first-born children are more likely to have higher blood pressure later.

How do such effects come about? They relate to a phenomenon known as 'maternal constraint'. To understand it we need to think back to our evolutionary past. We represent the result of a compromise. We evolved from a quadrupedal into a bipedal primate—in other words, into walking upright—somewhere in East Africa about 5 million years ago when we left the forests and entered the savannah. We can only speculate about the reasons why our distant ancestors started to walk upright. It may have been that it conferred advantages in a savannah setting where it was possible to see further and to run around. Indeed, the human lineage has the only primates that can run for very long distances—as every charity knows that encourages us to run marathons. We cannot, of course, run as fast as the big cats or other predators which might have attacked us, or as fast as the antelopes or other large mammals which might have been our prey. But because we can run for long distances we are able to run these animals to exhaustion if we work as a team, rather like in a relay race. This may have been one of the critical advantages in allowing us to survive in the savannah environment. But running requires a narrower pelvis, otherwise we would just waddle. So the human pelvis evolved to be narrower than that of other primates.

And there are also other problems with standing on two legs. In non-human primates such as gorillas, and even our closest cousins the chimpanzees, the abdominal contents hang downwards as they walk on all fours. This is not inconvenient and does not compromise digestion. However, in the upright position the intestines will tend to descend into the lower abdomen and be squashed into the pelvis. If the muscles of the pelvic floor are not to be used continuously to support them, then the shape as well as the size of the pelvis needs to be modified. So the width of the pelvic canal narrowed substantially, over thousands of generations of selection. The angle of the pelvic girdle, to which our legs are attached, has also rotated—we can see the difference very easily if we look at the way that the legs of a dog or a cat, or for that matter a cow or a horse, are attached. It is very hard for them to walk on only their hind legs.

But now consider the implications of this during the birth process. The fetus must pass through the pelvic canal from the mother's womb during birth. And as the human pelvic canal is significantly narrower than that of the chimpanzee, our nearest cousin, the birth process is much more difficult. And it's harder still because humans have evolved to have much larger brains, and therefore much larger skulls to hold them, than any of our primate relatives. This rapid brain growth starts before birth, and is not completed until after birth—otherwise we could never be born through that narrow pelvic canal at all. Our brains are much more immature at birth compared to our monkey cousins—we are born comparatively helpless and unable to move around.

For the large head of the human baby to pass through the narrow pelvic canal is challenging. Indeed, that is why humans are the only animals for which some form of birth assistance is generally required during the natural process of giving birth. Perhaps it is no surprise that in the absence of modern medical care obstructed labour, where the fetus literally becomes stuck and delivery cannot progress, is, sadly, a relatively common problem. In some undeveloped societies up to 60 in every 1,000 births encounter this problem.

We can see the extent of this problem if we return to our ancestral homeland in the Rift Valley. In the highland plains of what is now Ethiopia, women of the Hansa or Mursi tribes are only too aware of the problem of obstructed labour and its disastrous consequences. The tremendous contractions of the uterus during labour, in order to force the fetus through the pelvic canal, can tear the women's internal organs and produce a rupture—a fistula—which may rip her urinary tract or her rectum. Such labours can go on not just for many hours but for many days, and when this happens very often the fetus dies. Often the mother will die as well.

It may take the woman several days to reach hospital and she will probably not start the journey until obstructed labour is clearly a problem. Despite the agony of the labour and the wrenching obstruction, she may have to walk for more than a day to reach the nearest road, and then possibly travel on a truck for another day to reach the nearest city. By this time the fetus is almost certainly dead, and all that the doctors can do is deliver it and try to repair the woman's reproductive tract. Up and down Ethiopia, hospitals have been set up—initially by missionaries like Catherine and Reginald Hamlin in the 1960s—and since the establishment of these hospitals, 35,000 women have been treated for reproductive tract fistulas. Many more never made it to hospital—and consequently, they suffer from urinary or faecal incontinence and often live in shame and social isolation.

We have to note here that this problem is made worse by the practice of female genital mutilation. Some groups, in Ethiopia and other parts of the world, demand female circumcision—something we find abhorrent in the West. The scars themselves narrow the opening of the vagina but frequently it is also sewn up, leaving only a very small opening. If this ligature is not removed before labour, the consequences can be dire.

Under rural conditions there is not very much that can be done about the problem of obstructed labour, although having a friend or relative to assist during the delivery process can help. There are also, of course, many folk remedies and other fables about what a woman might do to reduce the risk of obstructed labour, usually based on the idea that having a smaller baby will help. Undoubtedly this is true—but, as we have seen, the fetus has a surprising amount of control over its own growth. So Ethiopian women who refuse to drink milk during pregnancy, perhaps to reduce their calcium intake and so reduce the growth of the fetal skeleton, may not actually reduce their risk of obstructed labour, even though they will increase the risk of rickets in their offspring.

Obstructed labour would have been a disaster in our Palaeolithic past. We can imagine that it would have been common for big males to mate relatively juvenile girls. Many of the girls who had a fast-growing male fetus would have died in obstructive labour. So now might evolution have helped to protect us against this problem?

It turns out that the growth of every fetus is, to a certain extent, constrained by its mother; this helps to match its size at birth to the size of her pelvis. This means that the mother's physiology and metabolism will control the growth of the fetus rather more than its genes, which of course have been partly inherited from the father. There could be a major conflict if the genetic component from a tall male had combined with that of a small female to produce the next generation. A pregnancy involving an especially large fetus develop-ing in the womb of a relatively small woman would be far more likely to end in disaster. This is where the maternal constraint of growth exerts its most powerful effects.

Humans are not the only animals in which this process has been observed. The first demonstration was published in 1938 by Arthur Walton and John Hammond. These researchers crossed small Shet-land ponies with the large shire horse breed traditionally used to pull the plough, and then looked at the size of the foals born. When the mare was a Shetland pony and the sire was a shire horse, the size of the foal was much closer to that of a Shetland foal. Conversely, when the mare was a shire horse, the foal was nearly as large as a shire foal, even if the father was a Shetland pony. Needless to say, these experiments were conducted using artificial insemination.

When we look back at Walton and Hammond's original experiments, it seems surprising to modern scientists that they were ever published, as the number of animals used was relatively small even if the results were decisive. However, the experiments have recently been repeated in Cambridge by Twink Allen and Abigail Fowden using embryo transfer, and once again it is clear that these powerful processes operate in horses.

More recent observations in relation to humans have studied what happens in surrogate motherhood. Where an embryo is donated by one woman to another, and thus develops in the uterus of the second woman, the fetus born is closer in size to other children of the recipient mother than to those of the donor mother. So it seems clear that the mother's intrauterine environment is more important, in this case, than the genetic make-up of the fetus.

The degree of constraint can vary, and is greater in the first pregnancy in a woman's life. This makes sense in evolutionary terms because a woman's pelvis does not reach maximal width until four years after her first period. In the past it was inevitable that she would have been pregnant well before then—fertility is usually good two years after the first period. The underlying mechanism may involve the blood vessels supplying the uterus, which normally dilate and increase their flow during pregnancy, but are not as conditioned to do so in the first pregnancy as in subsequent pregnancies. Another reason might be the sheer demands on resources which pregnancy makes. If the woman is a teenager and her body is still growing at the time that she becomes pregnant, the question arises of whether it would be better to devote those resources to her growth or to the growth of her baby. From an evolutionary point of view the answer is unequivocal—it is better for the resources to be used to grow the mother than her offspring. After all, even if the pregnancy fails she can become pregnant again, and this accords with the harsh but realistic evolutionary process.

So, on average, first-born children are about 100 g smaller than subsequent children. This may not sound like much, but remember that we are not focused on birth weight, but on the signals which the intrauterine environment might give the fetus so that it can predict its future nutritional environment, and birth weight is only a poor indicator of these signals.

Shorter mothers tend to have a smaller pelvis, so again maternal constraint is greater. In places like India where there are multiple generations of stunting due to inadequate childhood nutrition and infection, birth weights are much lower than we have come to expect in the West. The average birth weight in some parts of India might only be 2,600 g—a weight we would regard as being growth retarded in the West. Indeed the World Health Organization regards a birth weight of less that 2,500 g as being growth-retarded, but this would encompass 40 per cent of some Indian populations, many of whom may be nonetheless healthy at birth.

Women who have their first pregnancy after the age of 35 also tend to give birth to smaller babies. This is an increasing problem as more women choose to do so for economic or social reasons. And many of them need in vitro fertilization for, sadly, fertility is declining by that age. IVF is associated with a higher incidence of twins and this leads to greater maternal constraint. This is because there is a limit to how much nutrition the mother can deliver to her fetuses, so fetal development will be even more constrained with triplets or quadruplets.

Considering smaller family size, short mothers, elderly first-time mothers, and multiple pregnancies, not to mention maternal and placental disease, we can see that for many populations well over 70 per cent of fetuses are likely to have a constrained perception of the nutritional world ahead of them.

There are biological reasons why it is safer to predict living in a bad nutritional world after birth than a good one. First, as we saw in the Jamaican infants, being set up to predict a bad nutritional world may make us more likely to survive famine. For many years this was thought to be the main reason behind these processes, but it now looks less certain that our Palaeolithic ancestors had to deal with much famine. We now think that the processes are more subtle. Predicting a harsh world gave the offspring a tendency to lay down fat when they could. This is important as the large and growing human brain has a high demand for energy. It does not reach full size until about seven years of age, and by that time the Palaeolithic child would no doubt have been exposed to multiple episodes of diarrhoea and other infections. To be primed to lay down fat as an energy store would thus be helpful. Furthermore, mild to moderate adiposity promotes fertility. The problems that come from being set on a path of predicting a poor nutritional environment appear only later in life, and then only if we live in a nutritionally rich environment.

And that is the key point—prediction is fine if there is an approximate match between what is predicted and what happens. We say approximate because every one of us has flexibility in our metabolic capacities and copes quite well with a range of energy loads. But, as the rat experiments showed, the greater the degree of mismatch the more likely we are to suffer the consequences in terms of obesity and disease. The greater the degree of maternal constraint the greater the likelihood of mismatch, and the greater the richness of the world out there the greater the degree of mismatch. Indeed, it turns out that all those groups we discussed—first-born children, children born prematurely or growth-retarded, children who are twins, children whose mothers eat less than optimally—are generally all at greater risk of obesity, diabetes, and cardiovascular disease.

There are also some examples of mismatch driven by human behaviour. Smoking reduces the passage of essential nutrients such as amino acids across the placenta to the fetus, and some environmental toxins can do the same. Excessive exercise in pregnancy can affect fetal nutrition too. There is some evidence that bottle-feeding increases mismatch and hence the risk of obesity later in life, because infant formula provides much more energy than breast milk. However, unbalanced modern diets can also affect breast milk quality, and this is an area about which we do not have much information and where more research is urgently needed.

Because diabetes and cardiovascular disease have insidious onsets, the greater the mismatch the earlier in life the clinical disease is manifested. We can see now how the graded relationship between birth size and disease risk is established. While maternal constraint does not lead to abnormal fetal growth retardation, it may subtly affect growth within the normal birth weight range, and thus affect later risk.

Moving for good?

There is another way in which mismatch occurs.

Humans move—they migrate and change their habitats. We have done this as a species from the time that our ancestors migrated out of Africa about 70,000 years ago, but the modern world has seen more migration than ever before. Some was forced—particularly by the slave trade and by the consequences of colonization and warfare. Much was voluntary, although economic or political in origin: the many thousands of Italians who travelled to the USA at the end of the 19th century and the beginning of the 20th century to seek a better life, the immigrants from Puerto Rico and many other Hispanic countries who moved to North America, the evacuation of the Falasha Jews from Ethiopia to Israel, and more recently the movements of people from eastern to western Europe and from North Africa to Italy. Nearly always these people are moving from a poor environment where they may be persecuted, under-nourished, or exploited, to a land in which they hope there will be more security and better education and healthcare. And everywhere people move from the countryside to the city. For the first time in our history more people now live in cities than in rural areas. They too come hoping for employment, for their children to get a better education, and to be better connected to modern society.

We say 'hoping' because very often their dreams are not fulfilled. All too often people migrating from low-income parts of the world to supposedly higher-income parts end up as the urban poor in their new homes—from the frying pan into the fire. This is clearly the situation in many parts of India where every month thousands of rural poor move to the cities in search of a better life.

Think of two brothers from rural Maharashtra who move to Mumbai and manage to raise a loan to buy an auto-rickshaw. They hope they will soon be sufficiently well-off financially to bring their families from the country too. It does not work out. After many months they decide that their wives should move to Mumbai, to assist with the cooking and washing and possibly to take on some outworking at home. They become ensconced in one of the slum areas of Mumbai. In time, several children are born. Another family has been established in a cycle of disadvantage and poverty. In the process, their lifestyles and those of their children have changed dramatically. The hard physical labour of working on a subsistence farm in the countryside is now replaced by sitting in a rickshaw in heavily polluted traffic or at home over a sewing machine in bad light. The city diet is rich in fat and sugar and salt as fast food outlets are the easiest way to eat during a busy working day—although it's pan puri here rather than McDonald's. Even the kind of fat consumed has changed. In the country, the diet would be low in fat apart from wedding and feast day food cooked in ghee, made from clarified butter. In the city, the oil in which much of the food is fried is a metabolically dangerous hydrogenated fat of questionable industrial origin.

The educational system or healthcare system in many slums on the edge of cities is no better than it was in the country. We can easily see how the biology of the woman born in rural India, of short stature, thin, and with a relatively small womb and pelvis, can give birth to a child who is totally mismatched to the life of urban Mumbai or Kolkata. These processes can explain the rapid increase in obesity among children which has occurred over a generation in migrants and where there have been rapid changes in diet and lifestyle through the developing world. The effects are just as dramatic—or more so—as those resulting from increased affluence in parts of the developed world.

A terrible tragedy is unfolding in parts of the South Asian subcontinent—as it is across China, Africa, and South America. Increasingly the mismatch which accompanies the rapid shift to a Western lifestyle, usually within a generation, is producing a wave of young people with obesity, and changes in their biology have put them on the path to diabetes or heart disease, if indeed they do not already suffer from them. These people may have to take drugs for the treatment of these conditions for the rest of their lives—if they can afford it—and slowly but surely the diabetes and circulatory problems will take a toll on many organs in their bodies. It will reduce kidney function, which means that an increasing number of them will go into renal failure and may need dialysis or kidney transplants. These are expensive and there is a limited source of donors, so many of them will die. The problem has also fuelled an illegal trade in organs—from donors (or their families acting for them!) who have 'donated' a kidney for cash.

The problems do not stop at the kidney. Diabetes will affect the blood vessels in many of the muscles in the body, making it hard for the person to exercise and even to look after themselves. The poor blood supply, especially to their lower limbs, will lead to ulcers, infections, and a high risk of needing an amputation. The diabetes will affect the little blood vessels supplying the retina of the eye, leading to blindness. This situation is getting worse by the year and it is calculated that by 2030 the number of diabetics in India will reach nearly 80 million.

The health costs of the condition will be enormous. All this in a country that cannot afford to vaccinate all its children against life-threatening diseases such as polio, measles, and whooping cough—single-shot vaccinations which cost a few dollars and give lifelong protection. How can such societies afford high-cost medical therapies for such a large part of the population?

And the challenge is no different in China, Indonesia, Mexico, Brazil, or the Gulf states . . .

Both thin and fat

We may have answered the question of why a poor start to life can lead to a greater risk of developing diabetes and cardiovascular disease, but to be able to stop the problem we have to have a clear idea of the biological processes that lead to this.

The first clues to answering this question come from India itself. Consider the babies born there: they are small babies but not necessarily thin babies. Even if they look thin they may have more fat on board than might otherwise be expected. Chittaranjan Yajnik is a renowned diabetes specialist in Pune, a city about 100 miles inland from Mumbai. Some years ago he started to make some simple measurements of the sizes and shapes of Indian babies at birth, analysing (with new scanning techniques as they became available) the composition of their bodies and comparing them to that of babies born of white parents in the UK. As we have already described, Indian babies tend to be smaller than European white babies, weighing almost 600 g less on average at birth. The surprising finding was that these babies were not equally small in every aspect of their bodies. They had relatively less skeletal muscle in their bodies and relatively more fat than their European counterparts. This fat was not under the skin but largely inside their abdomens, the visceral fat we described earlier as being most associated with later disease. Yajnik called this the 'thin outside-fat inside' baby.

Putting our evolutionary ideas into the story, we can see that this is a sensible body composition for these babies. If we predict a nutritionally limited future, we invest less in growth of metabolically active tissue like muscle and lay down more fat in order to have an energy reserve for when it is needed.

If the situation of the thin-fat Indian baby indeed represents normal biology—and we think it does as part of a response of the fetus to the conditions of prenatal life—then we might expect to find such variations even in Western babies. They may not be so obvious, but they should be there.

This is precisely what has been found in Southampton Women's Survey babies. Guttorm Haugen and Torvid Kiserud are obstetricians from Norway who worked with the Southampton investigators using advanced ultrasound techniques to study the way that blood flows around the fetal body in late gestation. In women who were relatively thin and who consumed an unbalanced diet—high in red meat, sugar, crisps, cakes, and white bread, but low in fruit and vegetables—the patterns of blood flow were different from those in fetuses whose mothers consumed a healthy, balanced diet. The amount of blood coming back from the placenta and going to the fetal liver was increased, and the amount going to the developing fetal heart and brain was correspondingly reduced. And this pattern of blood flow was associated with greater fat in the babies at birth—they seemed to be like the thin-fat Indian babies. Subsequent studies have shown that this difference is still present in the same children at the age of four, so it appears that the trajectory of fat deposition which starts before birth continues throughout infancy and early childhood.

Digging deeper

But we need to go down another layer in explaining the mechanisms of how a less than optimal start to life has long-term consequences. To do this excavation, we must use the techniques of molecular biology. We inherit the genes in our DNA from our parents but, as we explained earlier, next to the genes are segments of DNA that control gene function itself. These control regions can be envisaged as panels of switches—switches that tell genes when to be turned on and when to be turned off. For example, the insulin gene is turned on in pancreatic cells but as the settings are specific to cell types, the insulin gene will be turned off in liver cells.

Some switches are on or off at different times in life. So while the DNA sequence we inherit does not change during life, the switches controlling genes can be biochemically altered—as we go through puberty or old age, for example. But most importantly, these switches can be set to on or off in response to environmental signals received in early development. These control processes are complex because there can be thousands of these switches on every gene. They respond to molecules called transcription factors, which are the signal for turning the genes on and off and, because they are made by yet other genes, we end up with a very complex network of fine controls in every cell which use all sorts of feedback loops. But while changes in gene control can be very subtle, they can nonetheless have major effects.

These gene switch states are most modifiable in early development. This can be achieved by some chemical modifications such as methylating specific parts of the DNA—a surprisingly simple change which involves merely adding one carbon and three hydrogen atoms to a receptive site on the DNA. Other changes affect the histones—protein cores around which the DNA is wrapped and packaged and which are necessary to allow the approximately 2 m of DNA in every cell to be packaged into a small space. These are very carefully regulated steps in cell biology and we call them epigenetic changes. Epigenetic changes are passed from one cell to its daughter cells when it divides. As we develop from a one-cell embryo into a complex being, we start differentiating into various types of cells and these have different types of epigenetic profiles in them. Epigenetic mechanisms play a critical role in many biological processes—for example, they stop certain types of viruses that got incorporated into our ancestors' DNA from being active in us. Another function is to silence one of the two X chromosomes in every female cell so that the female does not get twice the dose of gene expression compared to males, who have only one X chromosome in each cell.

One of the most exciting discoveries in developmental biology has been that developmental plasticity depends on epigenetic processes. For example, the queen bee and the worker bee are both female bees; the only difference is that they have different epigenetic states, and we now know that these different states are induced early in life by what the larva is fed by the drones as it develops.

In recent years it has become possible to measure each individual gene switch by sophisticated molecular techniques, often using very expensive equipment. So, if our ideas are right we should find epigenetic changes associated with altered fetal experiences, and these might be related to what later happened to the offspring—especially in relation to disease risk. With this in mind, we decided to look for DNA methylation changes in very precise bits of the gene regulatory regions. We started searching in rats, while other groups around the world embarked on similar studies. Irrespective of how a poor start to life was induced, whether by changing maternal nutrition, or by giving the mother high doses of a stress hormone, changes in these gene switches were found in many important places in the DNA of the offspring. They were quite specific, however, occurring not randomly throughout the DNA, but on genes where the setting of the switch could have quite major consequences.

One set of experiments was particularly revealing. Michael Meaney, a neuroscientist in Montreal, used a well-established experimental model, in which he compared the offspring of rats that were well cared for with those poorly cared for by their mothers. How 'good' a rat mother is in looking after her young pups is indicated by how much licking and grooming she gives them. Those offspring that were poorly looked after grew up to be anxious animals, with high stress hormone levels in their blood-stream and, if they were female, became poor mothers themselves. By experiments in which he fostered pups onto different mothers he was able to show that this was not a genetic effect, but was set up by the early life experience. Meaney found that the effect was due to the triggering of an epigenetic change in a hormone receptor in the brain—indeed in the very receptor and the very pathway which would lead to high stress hormone levels. Lastly he used a drug which undid the epigenetic change and showed that it reversed the gene switch change and, even though the offspring were now adults, their behaviour returned to normal. Here was the proof that early, developmentally induced epigenetic changes could have life-long effects on behaviour.

At the same time, Karen Lillycrop and Graham Burdge in South-ampton were studying the effects of the diet fed to pregnant rats on epigenetic processes in their offspring. Using a diet low in protein and high in carbohydrates, they found that the pups showed epige-netic changes not only in stress hormone receptors but in the gene pathways controlling metabolism of fats in their livers. Just as in Meaney's experiments, the effects seemed to be permanent in the adult offspring. But, once again, it was possible to prevent them by giving an additional nutritional stimulus during development—here it was the micronutrient folic acid, and the cancelling effect occurred even though the pregnant animals were still on the low-protein, high-carbohydrate diet.

Inspired by this study, we studied Mark Vickers' rats that had been given leptin—these are the rats that had been tricked in their prediction and did not get fat, pre-diabetic, or eat to excess when given a high-fat diet. Leptin not only stopped the animals developing obesity; it stopped them having the epigenetic changes induced by prenatal under-nutrition. And Rebecca Simmons, a neonatologist in Philadelphia, used a different rat model of a poor start to life in which she found that giving newborn rats a drug related to a hormone made by the stomach reversed the abnormalities in the insulin-secreting cells of pancreas as well as the epigenetic changes in a gene controlling pancreas development.

These experiments make a compelling case that epigenetic processes are involved in the predictions which fetuses and infants make about their future lives, based on cues from the mother. This is a rapidly moving field—there is now a flood of studies showing epigenetic changes in animals which support these ideas.

Cutting the cord

As so often in experimental medicine, studies in animals reveal the important questions to ask in humans. As yet the human epigenetic data are more limited. There are some data suggesting that survivors of the Dutch Hunger Winter have changes in gene switches which can be seen in their white blood cells as adults, but the effects are small and the data difficult to interpret. Because white blood cells are made all the time, it is hard to relate epigenetic changes in them (in an adult) to a person's early development. What was needed was a source of DNA collected from the person as a fetus which could be related to that person's characteristics later.

It turned out that by good fortune or foresight, in the Southampton cohort studies umbilical cord tissue had been collected and deep-frozen at birth to preserve it. This provided a source of DNA to study. Combining the forces and resources of our laboratories in Auckland and Southampton, we decided to measure the gene switches in this DNA. Our molecular biologists, led by Karen Lillycrop and Allan Sheppard, had to develop new techniques to do so, and given the implications of anything we might find, we had to be very careful and pedantic with our methodology.

We did indeed find some gene switch changes that were associated with birth weight but these were not what interested us most. We wanted to know whether we could prove that developmental influence had important lifelong echoes even for children within the normal birth weight range because, as we discussed earlier, the risk of diabetes and cardiovascular disease is graded across the normal range. So if epigenetic changes are associated with this risk we should pick them up in normal weight babies.

The Southampton children have been followed for some years and have been extensively studied. They have had scans to measure the amount of fat and muscle and the density of bone in their bodies; they have had intensive cardiovascular measurements made; they have been examined for allergic outcomes; and they have even had cognitive and behavioural tests performed. So we set out to look for relationships between epigenetic changes at birth and measures of disease risk later in childhood. What we found astonished us.

First we looked at body composition. In our first study we found that the degree of epigenetic change measured at birth in one particular gene, associated with the control of fat metabolism, explained about 25 per cent of the differences in body fat between children nine years later. These results astounded us but we were nervous. The nature of science is such that extraordinary results can be an accident or a fluke. Therefore the more outlandish the result, the more important it is to replicate it. And for us this was an extraordinary result, maybe the most important of our careers—if it was right. It suggested that just measuring one gene switch at birth could tell us far more about which person might develop obesity than all the billions of dollars spent on looking at structural mutations in genes had found. If this result was true it had two enormous implications: firstly, that the developmental period before birth was far more important in determining risk of obesity than most researchers and doctors had expected; secondly, it shifted the focus for future research from genomic variation studies following the Human Genome Project to epigenetic processes. We had to find out whether this first result was right or not.

So we repeated the study—not once, but twice, using a second birth cohort—the famous Southampton Women's Survey we described before. The results were identical to those in the initial study. Methylation changes at birth in one particular gene at one particular site tell us much more about whether or not children will get obese than genetic variation.

And the work led to another important conclusion. We were able to show that the epigenetic switches measurable in the child's umbilical cord after birth were related to the mother's diet in early pregnancy. We showed that the switch was in the healthier direction in babies of women with higher carbohydrate and lower dairy protein intakes. We do not yet know how this comes about, let alone the answer to the *why* question that we flagged up earlier in the book, because association does not prove causation. It may be that it is some other aspect of the woman's diet or lifestyle associated with carbohydrate intake that is important.

When the work was published in the journal *Diabetes*, journalists wanted to know what this meant for mothers' diets. Unfortunately we cannot yet answer this fully, as it would be unsafe to go beyond the current data to be more precise. But with this knowledge we can now start evaluating which diets before and during pregnancy produce the best epigenetic profiles in the babies and thus the most healthy lives as they grow up. This will be the next phase of our work.

And our work has thrown up other tantalizing associations. We have found epigenetic signatures that are reflected in altered bone density, which is important because lower bone density starts one on the path to osteoporosis, to altered blood vessel function, to increased risks of allergy, and to altered attention and behaviour. This fits very well with the animal data, but as yet we have not replicated and confirmed these findings. Once we have we will publish them.

But it is clear that life before birth has an enormous influence on one's destiny. Far more so than nearly everyone would have imagined. And life before birth can be influenced by what the mother does, working through epigenetic mechanisms to change the destiny of the child.

Through a new lens

The focus has shifted: we can now see that human development has a critical influence on the risk of developing obesity, diabetes, and cardiovascular disease and probably on many other aspects of what makes us what we are. Now we can begin to see how our parents affect that development, although it is not through the genetic mechanism which the Human Genome Project had hoped to reveal (but did not). Rather, our developmental environment affects epigenetic gene switches which are set in expectation of the world in which we predict that we will live later. These processes appear to have evolved so that the prediction can change aspects of our bodies to maximize our survival until reproductive age, and reproductive fitness itself. The mismatches of our modern world, and our longer lives, have now made the epigenetic switches inappropriate, resulting in a greater risk of disease. With this information we can predict with greater certainty than ever before the likelihood that a child will become obese, and so be on the risky road to diabetes or cardiovascular disease.

The implications are broader than just having new knowledge. As epigenetic measurements become more established we can use that information in many ways. We can use it in research to find out what mothers should do to get the best outcomes for their pregnancies. We can use it to predict the probable destiny of tomorrow's children, and we can then use it to see whether various ways of bringing up our children—what and how we feed them, for example—might give them the healthiest possible destiny.

Dads matter too

We can imagine (and we know from experience!) that about half of those reading this will be somewhat annoyed, maybe even a little angry, about this. Are we saying that what happens to us is all our mother's fault? That the responsibility for chronic disease, and the solution to it and the blame for it too rest entirely with women?

We are most definitely not, for two reasons ...

Firstly, much of the variation in fetal experience that causes epigenetic change is likely to be subtle. Mothers can do nothing, for example, about their height, or whether this is their first pregnancy, so any idea of blame is completely inappropriate. However, with the new knowledge we are gaining we can develop much better advice for mothers about how they should care for themselves and their developing fetus during pregnancy. Current advice is not good and better advice is badly needed. We will return to this point.

Secondly, fathers do really matter too. While the results are only just starting to emerge, there is enough experimental data coming from studies in rats and mice to show that fathers can transmit signals through their sperm which also affect their baby's epigenetic state. Certainly, fat or stressed male rats can father offspring who become insulin-resistant or obese. And from studies using chemical toxins we know that epigenetic changes can be transmitted from one generation to the next through sperm.

We are just beginning to scratch the surface of the science here, but it is safe to say that what either parent does might affect their offspring. We know more about the maternal effects and it is inevitable that the mother has a greater influence—through the months of pregnancy and nursing, if not for any other reason. But if we are to help the next generation to be healthier by improving their developmental environment, we must enlist the help of both parents, and not blame either of them for processes which are all part of the nature of being human.

9

Taking Sugar

Toxic fat

Mothers are changing—many are getting fatter and more and more women suffer from a transient form of diabetes during pregnancy. Can these changes also contribute to the risk of diabetes and heart disease in the next generation? There is compelling evidence that they do.

Maternal obesity is now a major concern and the focus of much recent investigation. This has shown that women who are obese are more likely to give birth to babies who themselves will become obese as children. All the signs suggest that these children will go on to have a higher risk of diabetes and cardiovascular disease.

The big question is—why? Why doesn't each generation start afresh, only becoming obese if its members consume excess energy or do not exercise enough? After all, this is the implication of the widely championed argument that these are the most important risk factors for obesity. Its advocates would argue that it is simply that people born into families where other members are obese learn the same habits of gluttony and sloth as their parents. Clearly children do learn from their parents and pick up exercise and feeding habits very early in life. In fact, that is a major argument for giving greater emphasis to early life as a point for intervention.

But there is more to it than this—in animal experiments conducted in many research centres it has been shown that giving high-fat diets to pregnant animals leads to the mothers giving birth to pups which themselves become fat. For example, when Maqsood Elahi and Felino Cagampang in Southampton fed female mice a high-fat diet from the time of puberty, they gained weight, and interestingly their offspring ate more, exercised less, had high blood pressure, became fat, and showed inflammatory markers in their blood—they looked very much like humans with the metabolic syndrome. The effects were worse if the offspring were also given the same high-fat diet as their mothers. As Kim Bruce and Christopher Byrne showed, these offspring laid down more fat in tissues such as the liver, so it seemed as if they had been primed to make the most of a high-fat diet, although if given it continuously they became sick. The parallels with the human condition are striking. Deborah Sloboda and Mark Vickers made similar observations in rats in Auckland and found almost identical results. For example, they fed female rats high doses of fructose, the sugar found in soft drinks, and showed that the offspring had unhealthy livers.

These effects, produced by feeding a high-fat diet to a pregnant rat or mouse, cannot be due to learnt behaviour or to genetic factors. The 'obesity begets obesity' phenomenon is yet another demonstration of the impact of development, of very early life experiences, in establishing our metabolic control and risk of disease.

But that still does not answer the *why* question: why is it that we have evolved with a biology such that when our mothers eat a high-fat diet we have a great risk of becoming fat and getting diabetes? And as we saw in the last chapter, we might also have some additional risk when our fathers are obese.

The first point to make is that parental obesity and exposure to very high-fat diets is not likely to be something our forebears experienced very often. Through most of our evolutionary history we were probably relatively lean and rarely had much access to high-fat foods. Some individuals may have become obese but they would have been rare. Accordingly we never evolved to cope with exposure to such high-fat foods and neither our maternal nor our fetal physiology is designed to deal properly with them. But how does this explain how obesity is passed on to the next generation?

We saw in the last chapter that a pregnant woman's consumption of an unbalanced diet—particularly one that signalled a poor nutritional world—was likely to lead to her fetus laying down more fat in its body. We believe that this evolved because it would have provided some survival advantage for the infant under predicted difficult and unreliable conditions after birth. In particular, having extra fat as a child provides a fuel reserve to feed the hungry and rapidly growing brain in infancy and childhood, especially after weaning when the risks of under-nutrition might be high—from infection, famine, conflict, etc.

Starting life poorly can lead to relative obesity later in life and many women who are obese do actually consume an unbalanced diet. Indeed, somewhat paradoxically, many infants born to obese women are slightly growth-retarded, reflecting this unbalanced nutrition or other problems of pregnancy. They have started on the pathway to obesity that we described in the last chapter. But how does this explain why the babies born to obese mothers, of normal or large size, go on to become obese?

Just how nasty is fat?

There are at least two ways of explaining the processes which are going on. As so often in science, they are probably both correct, but we do not know the circumstances under which each operates; they may even operate simultaneously.

The first, and most commonly held, idea is that the consumption of a high-fat diet by the mother literally produces toxic effects on her and on the placenta and so affects her growing fetus. These toxic effects build up as she becomes obese. The toxic processes in question involve free radicals, unstable molecules which use oxygen chemically to oxidize many components of the body, changing their function.

Exposure to a degree of such oxidative stress is a fact of life, because we make some free radicals all the time—it is a consequence of living in an atmosphere that contains 21 per cent oxygen. We cannot survive without it, even though, paradoxically, it is slowly killing us. Many of the processes of ageing are associated with the slow and inevitable damage from oxidative attack. However, the body uses a range of antioxidants, some enzymes, and vitamins C and E to destroy free radicals and limit this damage. But these systems can be easily overloaded. So it may be that excess fat leads to more free radicals which damage the placenta and its blood vessels, limiting nutrient supply to the fetus. The free radicals may even cross the placenta, attacking the fetal tissues directly. So this theory can certainly explain some of the evidence of damage seen in the placenta of obese humans and animals, and it can explain why some obese women give birth to babies that are smaller than average because of poor placental function. And so a pathway to developing obesity later is established.

We will discuss the second theory in more detail later in this chapter in relation to the diabetes of pregnancy. When excess energy gets to the fetus it can stimulate the fetus to make more insulin. Fetal insulin causes the developing fat cells to increase in number—so these babies are born with more fat cells. And if we start life with more fat cells, in the modern world they can become readily loaded with fat, and because we therefore have more capacity to store fat it becomes much easier to become obese.

An extension of this argument runs as follows. Some degree of body fatness is a good thing, and so if a mother is a little fat and is able to consume a rich diet, it might make evolutionary sense for her to signal to her offspring that the opportunity to capitalize on this environment exists. If a mother were able to indicate to her offspring during its development that it should look out for fat and sugar, and gobble it up when it can, this might have an advantage for the fetus in terms of its later reproductive (that is, evolutionary) success.

It *might*, we stress, because obviously the kinds of diets and lifestyle we now have are novel in evolutionary terms, so this process would only operate up to a certain point, almost certainly exceeded by now. But it can explain why the babies of some obese women go on to become obese themselves.

This idea fits with the biology of many other animals, especially those that breed at different times of the year, where it is essential for the metabolism of the offspring to be set from the time of birth or hatching if they are to get the most out of their environment. And it fits with some of the biochemical changes which we have found in organs such as muscle and liver of the rat and mouse offspring of fat-fed mothers, which appear to be more those of exaggerated normal function than of pathological dysfunction but which favour fat deposition. At first this is not harmful, and in fact it is part of an effective life-course strategy to promote greater reproductive success. But given the nutritionally rich world that many babies are now born into, these mechanisms soon lead to too much fat being laid down and damage to blood vessels and other cells, which put the growing child at risk of chronic disease.

Explanations derived from evolutionary biology are rather satisfying, but in this case the idea cannot really be tested except by extrapolation from animals. It does have implications, however, which we *can* test. One is that the processes by which a mother signals to her growing fetus information about aspects of her environment, including how obesogenic her diet is, might be expected to interact with those regulating fetal growth through the mechanisms of maternal constraint, which we described in the last chapter.

Now we can take the idea further. If, at the other end of the dietary and body composition spectrum, aspects of the mother's high-fat diet and adiposity are signalled to the fetus, then not only should the offspring of fatter women be more likely to become fatter as they grow up, but the first-born offspring of obese women should be the fattest of all as young adults. This is exactly what has been found in the Motherwell study that we described in the last chapter, where the first-born children, who were now adults, of obese women had a higher percentage of body fat than their later siblings. Importantly this interaction was seen across the entire range of levels of fatness in mothers from the thin to the obese—the fatter the mother, the fatter the offspring. There was no obvious cut-off in the level of maternal obesity at which pathology in the offspring sets in. This might argue that the toxic explanation we put forward earlier is less important than this evolutionary explanation. But either way, as so often in our story, we are in the territory of normal human biology within the normal range of human experiences, which is so overlooked and yet so important.

What about the father, though? If this theory about signalling nutritional states to the offspring is valid, could he not have a role too? Why leave it only to the mother to signal critical aspects of the environment to the offspring? One could expect the mother to have the dominant role, because mothers have a longer period of biological contact with their offspring during pregnancy and lactation, and because there were virtually no processes known by which the father could signal such things to his offspring anyway. His role was thought to be limited to what kinds of eating and lifestyle behaviours he might impart to his child as he or she grew up.

No one had really looked hard at this question until recently. But as we described briefly in the last chapter, a group from Australia has now shown that male rats that are fed to become obese sire offspring that have abnormal metabolic control as they grow up, regardless of the mother's diet and fatness. This suggests that in some way a signal is passed on in the sperm which influences the metabolism of the offspring. More than that we do not know at present—there is some data that epigenetic changes can be found in sperm and that these can influence the next generation. But whatever the mechanism, the implications for fathers-to-be are obvious. There is no room for complacency among males.

Sweet mums

We are facing a new epidemic—diabetes in pregnancy—and it is emerging with horrifying speed, particularly in some parts of Asia. This is a special form of diabetes—it appears in pregnant women, but then disappears after pregnancy. It will come back in the next pregnancy and in time most of these women will go on to develop diabetes even when they are not pregnant. Just 15 years ago the incidence of this transient diabetes in pregnancy—we call it gestational diabetes—was only about 7 per cent in places like Singapore. This is a percentage not very different from what we see in countries like New Zealand and the UK. But now more than 20 per cent of pregnant women in Singapore have gestational diabetes. The same rapid increase is happening in Hong Kong and China, where at least 20 per cent of women in the richer big cities now develop diabetes during pregnancy.

Diabetes in pregnancy has consequences for both fetuses and babies. If it is very severe, the placenta can be damaged and the fetus become severely growth-impaired or even die. Lesser degrees of gestational diabetes tend to do the opposite—they cause the fetus to grow bigger and this can override the constraining mechanisms we discussed in the last chapter. The fetus will lay down more muscle and, especially, more fat in its body. This is because glucose crosses the placenta easily; it means that when mothers have diabetes, they have high blood sugar levels and so then does their fetus. This leads the fetus to make more insulin, which leads it to make more fat cells. And because the fetus is receiving excess energy in the form of sugar, it then stores that excess energy as fat. The very biggest babies we see are those from diabetic mothers, and they can be so large that delivery is not possible without a Caesarean section.

But the babies not only become fat: they are also much more likely to develop diabetes themselves. Recently a large study has been carried out in over 2,300 Chinese people living in Hong Kong. About a quarter of those with diabetes had at least one diabetic parent and this was much more likely to be a diabetic mother than a diabetic father. This effect might have a genetic component, but as we have seen there is little evidence for this. And the fact that it is more commonly transmitted when the mother is the parent with diabetes points to a developmental factor. This is given strong support from the finding that people who developed diabetes were more likely to do so early if their mother had diabetes during pregnancy than if she developed it after they were born. Similar conclusions have been reached from a recent study with Canadian First Nations people, about one in five of whom will develop diabetes; up to a third of these cases can in turn be attributed to their mother having gestational diabetes.

Clearly, being in some way exposed to high levels of glucose as a fetus predisposes a person to develop diabetes later. The arguments have many similarities to those we presented above to explain how maternal obesity has effects on the offspring. Once again it is important to flag up the distinction between processes which are normal, even if they have consequences for risk of disease later, and those which are pathological from the start.

Early pregnancy is a finely balanced physiological situation where the developing embryo and its mother have to come to some agreement about the course ahead. More often than not they do not reach an agreement, because the majority of conceptions—as many as 70 per cent—end in early miscarriage. It may be that the balance between the immune system of the embryo and that of the mother is not right, and this of course will be critical for her to permit what is essentially a foreign being, with up to half its genes different from hers, growing in her womb for nine months. Or there may be other factors contributing to the incompatibility.

But despite what appears to be a somewhat unstable situation in early pregnancy, once implantation has been achieved and the placenta has been established to nourish the fetus, it actually becomes very hard to abort the fetus. History furnishes many examples of women involved in warfare, famine, flood, or earthquake in early pregnancy who yet successfully carry their fetuses to term. At this time in pregnancy the mother's resources must be optimally devoted to the development of the fetus—there is now no going back. This makes sense in evolutionary terms. The mother has invested a lot to ensure that her genes are transmitted to the next generation and it is more sensible to keep on investing than to start again. It is a dilemma that anyone who has started building or renovating a house knows well. Even if the architect and builder have grossly underestimated the cost, once you have invested so much you have little choice but to press on—returning to the bank manager yet again.

So why are mothers more likely to get diabetes in pregnancy? Yet again it is a consequence of what is a normal process becoming abnormal because we no longer live as we did thousands of years ago.

Glucose is the most important fuel for the human fetus and once the placenta has developed, it makes special hormones that change the mother's metabolism, helping to mobilize her own fat stores and to shift her biochemistry to one that consumes more fat and less glucose so that more of this sugar can pass on to her fetus. Even the protein stored in her muscles can be mobilized to provide essential amino acids so that the developing fetus can grow. These placental hormones change the mother's metabolism by inducing a level of insulin resistance—the state in which her own insulin works less well and akin, at a mild level, to what happens in diabetes.

But if the woman is herself already on the path to insulin resistance before she became pregnant, in pregnancy she is likely to become frankly diabetic—and this is gestational diabetes. We know that women who get gestational diabetes are more likely to develop diabetes even when they are not pregnant later in their lives, so there is clearly a connection, although it is pregnancy which seems to reveal the underlying problem.

There is a whole range of factors which contribute to women being at greater risk of developing gestational diabetes. Being overweight is one; eating a diet very high in fat and fructose during pregnancy is another. The hormones present during a pregnancy make a woman more sensitive to such a diet, and this effect is superimposed on any genetic and developmental factors that have already influenced her biology to set her risk of developing the condition.

Women who have a poor start to life, as well as those who had a mother with gestational diabetes, are more likely to get gestational diabetes themselves. Gestational diabetes is also more common in women suffering from polycystic ovarian syndrome, and this itself is more common in those who have a poor start to life. So there appear to be cycles of risk passed on from generation to generation by a range of processes.

It is clear that the early identification of diabetes, or potential diabetes, during pregnancy is of utmost importance, and that once identified it needs to be treated highly effectively. All too often doctors are satisfied to find a blood glucose level which appears to be within the normal range or is not too high at a particular point in time, rather than trying to track the day-by-day, and even hour-by-hour, variations in blood glucose in their patients. These swings in glucose can be quite dramatic even if the average level remains within the normal range. It may well be that it is, in fact, these swings that lead to adverse effects on the offspring.

Recent studies have shown that there is very little limit to the passage of glucose across the placenta from the mother to the fetus. This is in striking contrast to some other substances for which passage is clearly very carefully controlled by the placenta. It is almost as if the fetus cannot have too much of a good thing in the form of sugar.

It appears that evolution has led to the selection of mechanisms that defended our ancestors more against the risk of under-nourishing a fetus than of over-nourishing it. We believe that this is because the risk of over-nourishment was remote in times past. This lack of control might have had an advantage during evolutionary history by maximizing the nutrition of the fetus. Indeed because high-energy diets did not exist regularly in our evolutionary past and because, without modern medicine, gestational diabetes carries with it a high risk of fetal death, we would argue that gestational diabetes is not likely to have been a frequent occurrence during our evolution, so we have not evolved protective measures against it.

There is further evidence in support of this argument. The high levels of insulin resulting from the mother's high blood sugar mean that the baby also needs to run on high blood sugar after birth. This is unlikely to occur because most women do not find it possible to feed their infants abundantly soon after delivery. It is normal for it to take some days—on the first day the breast does not produce normal milk, but what is called colostrum, which is rich in immune proteins and hormones that are of great value to the baby's health. So blood glucose levels fall more dramatically in the newborn baby of a mother whose diabetes was not well controlled, driven by its high insulin levels, and this can lead to the brain being starved of glucose. The infant may become unconscious or brain damaged, or may even die. This is another reason why gestational diabetes would have been filtered out by evolution.

Starting life with more fat cells means that we have more fat cells for the whole of our life, because once made they stay with us. If we keep to a prudent diet these may not get loaded with fat but, as we have seen, it is hard to stay on a prudent diet in this energy-rich world. Later in life, having cells packed with fat leads to insulin resistance. But if we become insulin-resistant we have to make more insulin to get adequate amounts of glucose into our body's cells. At some point the pancreas cannot keep up with this increased demand to make insulin. So we cannot control blood sugar and in time we become diabetic.

Insulin resistance also leads to high blood fat levels and these fats enter the membranes of muscle and liver cells and change the way they work. This makes them more insulin-resistant still, and so the disease process is aggravated. It just gets worse and worse. So children who start life with more fat cells are more likely to get diabetes as they grow up, particularly in the kind of high food-energy world most of us now inhabit.

The key point is that these effects on the fetus are essentially adaptations of the developing organism to what it sees as a normal stimulus. The information it receives from its mother has consequences for its development. We are all, to a greater or lesser degree, adapted to the world in which our ancestors used to live and, as we saw in the last chapter, we try to use developmental plasticity in fetal life to adapt ourselves to the world we expect to live in as we grow up. But this is becoming harder and harder to do as the world that evolution designed us for is very different from the world of industrial agriculture, modern processed foods, and labour-saving devices.

The fat baby culture

We still think that a fat baby is a healthy baby, when in fact he or she may be on the path to obesity. It is obvious how this perception emerged. In the 19th century a thin baby was probably one who was under-nourished or growth-retarded and at greater risk of getting an infection, or just 'failing to thrive' as the phrase went among doctors of the period. Such babies were more likely to die. Measles and other common childhood illnesses could be death sentences for an under-nourished child, just as they are today in many developing countries. Sadly, several million children still die each year from under-nutrition and associated illnesses, particularly in Africa and parts of Asia. So as maternal and child health services emerged at the beginning of the 20th century, a key focus was on ensuring the adequate nutrition of infants. Specially designed infant formulas were developed and promoted at this time, which made it easy to provide infants with more calories than breast milk. So infants grew bigger.

In many parts of the world, bottle-feeding was marketed as socially desirable, convenient, and something which the modern, liberated woman and her partner should do. So, many women started to bottle-feed, and this did indeed help their babies to grow fat—but, regrettably, the beneficial effects of breastfeeding were lost. The tragedy of this emerged in Africa in the 1970s where aggressive marketing of infant formula led well-intentioned mothers to bottle- rather than breastfeed. As formula cannot provide the immune support that breast milk does, and the water used to make up the formula was often not clean, the consequence was epidemic gastroenteritis, which led to thousands of infant deaths. There are now very tight controls on the marketing of baby formula globally, and the major infant food companies generally act responsibly in this regard. Unfortunately this sense of responsibility is not universal, and smaller, nationally based companies can still break the rules—witness the recent tragedy in China where unscrupulous milk producers added melamine to the milk supply to trick buyers into thinking the milk had higher protein levels than it did—but melamine is toxic.

In middle-class Western societies, when women entered the workforce the use of infant formula also became more common. That breastfeeding might be compatible with women's rights is a very recent concept—but breastfeeding in the workplace is still uncommon and very often hard to maintain. We were slow to recognize the real health benefits of breastfeeding, and there is much more that needs to be done to make it easy and acceptable. We also now know that breastfeeding improves other aspects of the baby's life in addition to reducing the risk of chronic disease, including maternal–infant bonding, which can lead to improvements in brain development and behaviour.

So mothers and nurses grew up in the first half of the 20th century with the clear view that a fat baby was a healthy one. In the context of their times, that was probably largely correct. But the degrees of fatness have changed and the context of risk has altered dramatically. Just because a well-nourished baby is healthy does not mean that an over-nourished baby is more healthy—indeed he or she will certainly be less healthy in time. As we have seen, there are many reasons why a baby with excess fat may be on the pathway to future disease, but changing the mindset that a fat baby is a healthy baby will take time. Grandmothers might often chide their sons and daughters for allowing their children to be too thin when, provided they are growing, they are in fact fine. Far too many children in Western society are damaged by the baggage of this historically determined cultural perception.

Passing risk on

We have seen over the past two chapters that what happens in one generation can influence the next. It has been known for decades that women in the poorest circumstances, who have limited nutrition, give birth to children who become stunted. When their daughters grow up they will, in turn, will give birth to small babies. They will stay like this unless their world changes and energy-dense foods become available in large quantities. Then, as we described in the last chapter, their children are more likely to become mismatched and to be at risk of diabetes or cardiovascular disease. As some women start becoming obese their offspring are at greater risk. As time progresses some of these women will start developing gestational diabetes and yet another pathway to the intergenerational passage of disease risk is set up. In countries such as India, these various intergenerational pathways may operate at the same time. And even in the West, while emaciated mothers giving birth to children who become stunted adults are, thankfully, seldom seen, the other intergenerational pathways exist.

What are the implications of all this for the future? One important implication clearly concerns the mismatch between generations in term of diet. But surely, after the environmental transition has taken place, the situation should be relatively stable? Won't the increase in obesity and non-communicable disease, which has been so dramatic in many parts of the world, now begin to slow down? The *rate* of rise of childhood obesity is indeed now beginning to slow in some places, but it is still *rising*. Does this mean that we can be optimistic because, while we may perhaps have to suffer the consequences of childhood obesity for the next generation, things will be OK after that?

Unfortunately, as our research proceeds, we realize that the answer to this is clearly no. The various intergenerational pathways to transmission of obesity, diabetes, and cardiovascular disease will not disappear. Why should we think that we could change our biology, evolved over so many millennia, so quickly? Taken together, the many causes of a poor start to life and the growing incidence of gestational diabetes and maternal obesity make the implications very clear. The majority of children are likely to start life with increased risk of developing obesity and chronic disease.

Gestational diabetes appears to be a particularly dangerous feed-forward situation and it is emerging rapidly in some developing countries. There is no brake on this system—diabetes will beget diabetes and the rate of increase in gestational diabetes in Asia, as the nutritional transition proceeds, may lead to a situation where the majority of pregnancies will be complicated by it within a generation. Modelling of these intergenerational effects makes it seem inevitable.

Breaking this cycle is unlikely to be achieved by waiting until people develop diabetes; we must start thinking now about strategies that reduce the risk of gestational diabetes and its impact on the fetus. This has several components—it means focusing on the developmental factors that lead women to be at greater risk of metabolic compromise before and during pregnancy. We will discuss these strategies in the next two chapters. And it means managing gestational diabetes with much better nutritional education and support, in order to reduce the risk of high glucose levels attacking the fetus during pregnancy.

Reviewing the strategy

The question we pondered in earlier chapters is at least partially answered—our experience as embryo, fetus, and infant explains in no small part why some of us are more likely to become obese, and some are more at risk of diabetes and cardiovascular disease. Development is one missing piece of the puzzle and it is important to place it back into the picture.

When we are losing a war it is important to stand back and look at our strategy. Has the target been wrong, is the choice of weapons wrong, are we focused on winning one battle rather than adopting a long-term plan aimed at winning the war?

Some wars to promote health have been won. Think of the war on tobacco—while it is not a complete victory, we are winning it in most countries. In that case there was a simple enemy, one that could be removed—even if it turned out to be quite difficult to do so. There were the vested interests of the tobacco growers and the tobacco industry which had to be countered. There was the question of the large tax revenue from tobacco. There was much blurring of the evidence in order to create uncertainty as to whether tobacco really is harmful. There was the simple fact that many people are biologically addicted to tobacco products and that there are social and cultural contexts in which they smoke, which are not easy to change. But despite all this, after a long campaign, smoking is now restricted or illegal in many places in developed countries. Sadly and irresponsibly, the tobacco industry has turned its attention to the developing countries to boost its sales.

Why do people continue to smoke even in developed countries, where the information that it is harmful is widely disseminated?

For many it is a question of time preference. In their minds they discount the risks of later cancer or heart disease for the more immediate pleasures derived from nicotine and the social context that they share with other smokers. Some evolutionary psychologists such as Dan Nettle, whose work we described in Chapter 7, would argue that, particularly for people in poor communities, this discounting of the future is part of an even greater problem. In effect, they unconsciously predict a shorter life and therefore are less willing to invest for the future rather than live for the present. This might explain why smoking is more prevalent among poorer parts of Western societies—for them the future is now. It's another example of a life-course strategy, a trade-off, although here perhaps it has a social element.

We need to consider this argument because it also applies to life style and chronic diseases in general—poorer people are less willing or able to plan for the future. These are not decisions that are easy to change—they are inherent in the way our brains are constructed as a result of our evolution over many millennia—and we need to understand this context rather than just to put the blame on people in such situations. Understanding this should provide reasons for society to invest in these communities. David Sloan Wilson, a biologist who has applied evolutionary principles to studying neighbourhood health in Binghamton, a city in upstate New York, has shown that morbidity is reduced where neighbourhoods feel valued and supported. We might bear this in mind for the diseases we are focused upon in this book.

While targeting 'gluttony' and 'sloth' has been the focus of most public health initiatives, throughout this book we have pointed out that these may not be our real enemies in this war. There are many reasons why some of us cope better, and some worse, with the nutritional transition. Some of them lie in our genes, some in our social and cultural circumstances. But much starts in our development. We can do nothing about our genes, and tackling social and cultural issues takes much time and is a real challenge. Indeed, as we saw in the first part of this book, simple assumptions about how effective this tactic is can turn out to be wrong.

So our development stands out as an area for immediate attention. We have described the multiple pathways by which biological processes in early life can lead to a greater risk of diabetes and cardiovascular disease, and how these turn out to be much more important than we could have imagined even a decade ago. These reasons alone make development a key point for attention, but there are other reasons as well. Diabetes and cardiovascular disease are appearing at younger and younger ages in both the developed and developing worlds—so we must shift our focus to earlier points in our life-course if we are to prevent them.

In addition, we are beginning to understand how early life experiences influence food preference, appetite, and exercise motivation for the whole of life. How we want to eat and how we want to exercise are influenced by what happens in the first few years of life. And the epigenetic studies described in Chapter 8 demonstrate that we may be able to pick up markers of risk very early in life. With all this information we should be able to do *something*—what is holding us back?

10

Breaking Fate

The hangover

The morning of 1 January 2000—the champagne had gone flat in abandoned glasses and the last fireworks had smouldered out wherever they landed. The 21st century staggered to its feet, pretty much to take up where the last century had left off. But the evening just passed was not a celebration for everyone—it was really only an event for the Western world. Not everyone drinks champagne, or any other alcohol for that matter. Not everyone could afford to celebrate. Some had nothing to celebrate. Many did not even know that it was the start of a new millennium.

The headaches and tiredness weren't the only hangovers from which it would take time to recover. In 2000, the leaders of 189 nations and many international agencies had signed a declaration establishing the Millennium Development Goals, setting up targets aimed at improving the social and economic conditions in the poorest countries by 2015. They were all laudable initiatives that would improve the health and well-being of millions of people worldwide. Many of these initiatives were seriously overdue.

A number of the goals focused on women and children. For example, the third Millennium Development Goal aimed to eliminate gender disparity in primary and secondary education by 2005, and at all levels by 2015. The fourth goal aimed to reduce the child mortality rate by two-thirds and the fifth to reduce maternal deaths by three-quarters and to achieve, by 2015, universal access for all women to reproductive health.

Now it is more than a decade since those New Year parties. We can see that the Millennium Development Goals, like most other New Year resolutions, are going to be broken. While we have not yet reached 2015, it is clear that not a single one of the goals will be met, although a number of them were identified as needing urgent attention by a gathering of world leaders at the United Nations in September 2010, organized to take stock of the situation.

These issues have attracted wider attention too. Sarah Brown, the wife of the former UK Prime Minister, took up the cause of women's health. In an interview with the *Guardian* newspaper she said, 'If we can fix things for mothers—and we can—we can fix so many other things that are wrong in the world. Women are at the heart of every family, every nation. It is mostly mothers who make sure children are loved, fed, vaccinated, educated. You just can't build healthy, peaceful, prosperous societies without making life better for girls and women.' She was right even if, to a certain extent, this is stating the obvious. But action has been patchy and very much aimed at achieving the numerical goals themselves rather than improving the situation of women and children in general in many countries.

Indeed, perhaps as a result of the Millennium Development Goals, the major focus of international activity in the area of maternal and child health has actually narrowed. Because of the influence of a few opinion leaders, and particularly that of the dominant philanthropic foundation in this arena—the Bill and Melinda Gates Foundation—

much activity has become focused on a reduction in maternal and neonatal mortality. While this is important in itself, it ignores many of the other considerations about this important phase in our life-course, which can have many other longer-term consequences. Perhaps this is the trap of setting goals—they become ends in themselves, rather than being used as indices of a larger problem. No one would deny the urgent need to reduce the risk of maternal and neonatal death, but it is no less a concern to ensure that the children who do survive have the best chance to live healthy, productive lives.

It is easy to be critical but, while practical solutions seem apparent, we have to recognize that delivery remains a problem. This comes down partly to matters of cost and partly to societal attitudes in some communities which limit the priority given to women's and children's health. For example, when funds are available, the purchase of weapons and supporting the local political powerbase sometimes take priority over these basic needs.

Cultural change is needed if women are to be more empowered, so that they become pregnant at a time of their choice, a time that allows them to have completed their education, and receive adequate care during pregnancy. Too many women are not in a position to control critical aspects of their life, but the cultural issues are deep and very complex—look at Iran, Afghanistan, and many societies in Africa. Consider the consequences of female circumcision or of young girls forced into early marriage. We cannot impose Western ideals on other cultures, but equally, it is a shame that progress on matters concerning maternal health is so slow. Quite apart from the humanitarian issues, these practices slow economic development and the progression to social stability which all sections of the population want in many countries.

Returning to the question of maternal and infant mortality, we can see that the issues which underlie many of the Millennium Development Goals could be fixed if sufficient resources were available. Ensuring that well-trained midwives or birth assistants are present at births in the developing world, equipped with a sterile piece of cloth which can be used to tie off the umbilical cord and a sterile scalpel blade to cut that cord, will make a huge difference. An adequate supply of antibiotics will prevent the all too often fatal consequences of puerperal fever. A supply of clean water for those mothers who feed their infants with infant formula would prevent the two to three million infant deaths from diarrhoea that still occur every year.

Our millennium headache is far from over. And there is more to feel bad about. Not only will we fail to deliver on the Millennium Development Goals by 2015, but some of the major problems we face weren't even part of those goals. For example, the problems of adjusting to nutritional and socio-economic transition, which are the focus of this book, were not even mentioned.

New resolutions?

In 2011 the United Nations turned its attention to the non-communicable diseases and a high-level meeting of the General Assembly was held in New York. Some developing nations had urged that these diseases be included in a modified set of Millennium Development Goals but there was a consensus that this is not the way forward—we need action and progress more than symbolism. As the Director General of World Health Organization, Margaret Chan, put it, 'Why would we want to try to jump on a train that left the station ten years ago?'

Our concern is that a much more holistic approach is needed than has been demonstrated to date. We have focused our attention too much on the adult—too much on the simple assumption that it is feasible to shift people's eating and exercise habits and that, if this can be achieved, the challenge of obesity and chronic disease can be tackled. But clearly that is not so. As long as we keep our primary focus on the adult rather than adopting a much broader perspective, some gains may be possible but the war cannot be won. Until it is appreciated that there are both individual and population differences in our biological sensitivity to an increasingly obesogenic world, we cannot adopt the right tactical approach. This will require a culturally and socially appropriate approach for each society. It will require governments to get beyond the avoidance of their responsibilities by shifting the blame to individuals. And most of all it will require a much greater focus on 'development' in both meanings of the word.

Earlier in this book we described how difficult it has been to get the developmental perspective into the frame. It is worth asking why this is the case, because unless we understand that we cannot expect the situation to improve significantly. For despite the accumulation of such strong evidence, the role of development and its impact on disease continue to be seen as a marginal issue. Perhaps this will change soon—don't the enormously exciting data on the life-course and epigenetic contribution to disease risk create an imperative that cannot be ignored much longer? We would think so. Yet we are not optimistic. There remain many vested interests that may well keep the focus of effort on the adult rather than the child. There are many reasons why the developmental dimension is easy to ignore. If we are to make progress, we need to explore them.

Why has development been ignored?

The first reason is that it has been hard for many of us to see what can be done about the problem from the life-course perspective. Human development is seen as being too complicated. It is hidden from view, at least in the womb, and seen as being protected from external influences, good or bad. Development has been seen as encapsulated, separated from the world outside. But, as we have shown, this idea is completely wrong. The research over the past 25 years reveals without a doubt that the fetus can, and does, respond to external influences, and that its responses alter the course of development itself to set the risk of a range of later problems such as obesity.

We have seen how virtually every baby's metabolic fate is tied up in its experiences as a fetus: whether the mother is fat or thin, whether she has diabetes, whether she is dieting, whether she is young or old, whether it is her first baby, etc. And we have seen how new data suggest that this leads to changes in the epigenetic state of the offspring. And we have seen that some new and provocative data suggest that the father's lifestyle and physical state can also affect the offspring—it may well be that obese fathers have epigenetic changes in their sperm which pass on a greater risk of obesity and diabetes to their children. And there is growing evidence that interventions and actions in infancy and childhood can also have long-term benefits.

Given the mass of data, there is no longer any excuse for ignoring the importance of the beginning of life to our later health. Indeed the data we have reviewed about epigenetic gene switches at birth predicting whether a child is more or less likely to get obese are so compelling that it must shift the focus of prevention from the adult to the parent, fetus, and infant. The clinical, epidemiological, and experimental data all agree; the practical implications of the research discoveries showing that we start to face the modern world well before and soon after we are born can no longer be overlooked.

Prevention is always better than treatment. We now know that prevention must start before we are born and probably before we are conceived. The paradigm is very simple. While the molecular changes that start in our bodies before birth may be subtle, they change the way we will respond to the nutritionally rich world we will progressively face after we are weaned. Thus some people are set up early in life to be more or less likely to put on weight, to develop insulin resistance, or to have faulty blood vessels. Because they are more sensitive to the challenges of the modern world, the effects become greater and greater over time. It may only be a few hundred grams a year at first but over time frank obesity and its complications will develop. That is the insidious nature of this process and that is why it is generally too hard to intervene once the processes are clinically apparent. Our efforts must shift to the very beginning of life.

When we embarked on this research, we had suspected that this early phase of life was important and that it would involve most babies, not just the growth-retarded ones that the early researchers in this field had focused on. But frankly, we have been surprised by how important this effect seems to be—the studies on gene switches measured in the umbilical cords of babies from Southampton have shown the prenatal factors operating before birth to be much more important than we had imagined.

The neonatal and infant periods are also very important—breast-feeding for several months can make a difference to the later risk of obesity and disease. Both poor nutrition in infancy and excess nutrition, from the inappropriate use of infant formula and other foods, can have long-term effects. Paediatricians and nutritional scientists in London have shown that bottle-feeding can adversely affect intelligence later in life. Extreme under-nutrition in infancy impairs brain development. If it is followed later by better nutrition, this mismatch can set the child up to subsequently become obese and put him or her at risk of disease.

Unfortunately nutritional science has not received enough attention or support in the past few decades, while the search for the genetic basis of disease has taken prominence. So our knowledge of what constitutes optimal nutrition for the mother during pregnancy and lactation and for the infant after weaning is remarkably weak. Yet most research authorities believe that this work has already been done. They are wrong. They are caught in a mindset that nutritional research is old-fashioned and simply focuses on deficiencies and excesses. The new science of epigenetics changes this dramatically.

The recognition that epigenetic markers can be used to identify the effect of nutrition during pregnancy and probably also during infancy now gives us a way of moving forward. We can envisage trials, and are now planning them, where we can learn from the epigenetic state of babies what the best diet for the mother or the baby should be. We would imagine that over time this will be an enormously fruitful area. We may be able to develop foods for mothers while they are pregnant or lactating, and for babies after they are weaned, which are designed to produce the optimal epigenetic state and the lowest later risk of disease. This is not fanciful—while it may take a decade, early efforts in this direction have started.

As so often in biology, thinking about other species can give us insights into our own biology, or at least make us pause for thought and consider other ways of looking at our own bodies. Take marsupials for example. These intriguing animals diverged from our early mammalian ancestors about 150 million years ago. Unlike most mammals, they have a very primitive placenta and give birth to a very immature embryo which has to be nursed in the mother's pouch for many months before it can leave for even a few minutes. The wallaby's baby joey has at birth a simple sense of taste which allows it to crawl up onto a teat in the pouch—it is literally only 1 or 2 cm long at this stage and is extremely fragile. It does not even have fully formed lungs as yet, but can absorb oxygen through its immature skin which has no fur. It grows over the next few months fed entirely on its mother's milk. But this milk is quite remarkable, because it changes in its composition dramatically at different stages during the joey's development—one protein disappears, another appears, and there is a biochemical dialogue between mother and joey to provide the food it needs to optimize its development at a particular time.

Marsupials are very different from other forms of mammals because lactation has to do what the placenta does in most mammals—provide nutrients to embryo and fetus until it can start on its path to independent life. Because the joey's development in the pouch takes so long, while still suckling one joey the mother may give birth to another, much younger embryo, which also crawls up to reach a teat. Now there are two joeys in the pouch, of very different ages and maturity, and with very different requirements in terms of milk composition. Their demands are met by the mother producing a different type of milk from each of her teats—an apparently unique process in which these mammary glands respond to signals from the joey about its age.

These processes do not operate in humans, and in any case women cannot usually become pregnant while still lactating. This is an evolved mechanism which allows us to space our children out, as we know that infant mortality rises if human babies are born too close together. Marsupials have a very different strategy, based on having more offspring. But notwithstanding these differences, it is likely that there are many more subtleties to human milk than we understand. Human milk's composition does change over time. Colostrum, the thick product of the mammary gland soon after birth, is rich in proteins, hormones, and antibodies and has a critical role in establishing early immunity against infection. It is nothing like the milk that is produced once lactation is established and that too changes its composition as lactation progresses. Human milk contains hundreds of different molecules and not all women have the same mix. Could these different compositions play a role in influencing infant development? There might be a reason for this—perhaps an evolutionary one—but it is not yet known.

We know that whether a baby is fed on breast milk or formula from soon after birth changes the mix of bacteria that colonize the gut and we are beginning to realize how important that might be to future health. It is certainly another reason to promote breastfeeding. The mix of bacteria which is established in our gut in infancy essentially remains with us for life. One of the most exciting areas of medical research is using the power of modern molecular biology to sort out the thousands of strains of bacteria that inhabit our gut. Generally these bugs inside our bodies are very useful. They help by predigesting our food and play a major role in determining our nutrition and our metabolic health. We know that people with diabetes have different patterns of gut bacteria. We also know that how we develop this internal family of gut bacteria influences whether we get allergies—that is why many baby formulas and yoghurts for older people contain probiotics—strains of benign bacteria thought to be helpful and to promote health. In addition some milk products contain prebiotics—chemicals which are thought to enhance the growth of healthy bacteria.

Might it be that the mother's characteristics influence the composition of her breast milk more than we realize? A worrying trend is that as women become more obese the composition of their milk does indeed change. And over the past 20 years the ratio of omega-6 to omega-3 fatty acids in human breast milk has doubled, because many modern foods such as margarine and corn-fed meats contain high levels of the generally unhealthy omega-6 fats. From what we know about good and bad fats this is a worrying and unhealthy trend. The frightening implication is that human breast milk may well not be as healthy as it was a generation ago—even though it still provides clear advantages to the infant in terms of immune support and breastfeeding assists emotional bonding with the mother. Furthermore, because breastfeeding is driven by the baby, rather than by the mother's choice, or by practical matters such as the size of the teat on a feeding bottle, the risk of overfeeding is much lower. Generally, breastfed babies receive fewer calories than bottle-fed babies.

What happens during development may also play a major role in establishing food preferences and appetite later in life. We have seen how rats and humans who have been under-nourished early in life are more likely to require more calories to feel satiated later in life and that they prefer different foods, such as high-fat ones. These changes in appetite control appear to be associated with alterations to the wiring of the hypothalamus, the part of the brain which controls appetite.

Food preferences are informed by taste and smell. There are a limited number of distinct tastes we can detect, but we can distinguish between a wide range of flavours because we have a very large number of different cells in the brain system connected to our nose and palate. Between them, these smell and taste receptors give us the capacity to, on the one hand, savour a fine Bordeaux and make all sorts of comments on the intricacies of its bouquet and taste, yet reject rotten or unripe food on the other.

Human babies are born with a very limited number of tastes, in fact just two—sweet and salty. However, their palates can be broadened by the range of foods they are subsequently fed, and there is good evidence that what a baby is weaned onto, and how it is weaned, affect its later appetite control and food preferences. For example, repeated exposure to vegetables, even if they are initially disliked, can lead to greater acceptance of these foods over time.

There is also evidence that what a mother eats during pregnancy can lead to changes in her infant's food preference. For example, infants of mothers who drank carrot juice during pregnancy preferred carrot-flavoured cereals compared to those whose mothers did not consume any forms of carrot. Indeed, animal studies have shown that the mother's diet can change the balance of specific receptors in the brain which process odours. Furthermore, because flavours from food consumed by the mother can be directly reflected in her milk, maternal diet during lactation may also have an effect. Experiments have shown that exposure to flavours such as garlic through breastfeeding can determine the infant's eventual liking and acceptance of that flavour. So developmental exposures can influence eating behaviour in many ways.

We now know that in the first few years after birth, the brain circuits controlling energy regulation are established. These certainly include those related to appetite control and possibly also to exercise patterns. Whether these are hard-wired or are simply entrained behaviours that result from what the child has experienced is not entirely clear, but either way patterns for life are established very early.

There can be no doubt that the micro-world of the family that a baby is born into influences the way it grows up. If it is born into a family where excess eating is the norm, body image and behaviour will be affected. Food surveys have been done in many countries to see what babies are fed on. What these show is somewhat alarming. For example, French fries have become the most common vegetable given to infants in the United States. These studies consistently show that infants are being fed unhealthy, inappropriate diets with excess calories especially from fats and high-glycaemic-index sugars.

First-born babies may have a different biology owing to differences in the level of maternal constraint of their growth before they were born, but they are also treated differently. In Asia the sole child, especially a boy, is often called the 'little emperor', and his every whim is indulged by parents and grandparents.

Many attitudes passed down through generations date back to a time when illnesses such as gastroenteritis were common, and these limited the child's growth. So grandparents often have the attitude that a fat baby is a healthy baby—this is a belief that is no longer wise because the fat baby, at least in a Western country, is generally a baby at risk. In the West, how often does a person from the older generation express concern when a baby does not look chubby? The response of naive and concerned parents is almost inevitable and is often reflected in overfeeding and childhood obesity. Habits and perhaps their biological consequences are set up for life.

Yet not all such old-fashioned ideas are wrong. Take for example the concept of self-control. This is critical to adults in being able to manage their lifestyles—how to resist that extra cookie or to walk up two flights of stairs rather than take the elevator. There are many other aspects to self-control—control of emotions is a critical part of one's persona. Self-control is one of a number of higher skills, including social skills, task management, and impulse control, that are termed non-cognitive skills (cognitive skills relate to measures of intelligence). Work from developmental psychologists, and compiled by the Nobel laureate in economics James Heckman from Chicago, has shown that these non-cognitive capabilities are heavily influenced by the nature of upbringing in the first few years after birth. Vulnerable children from families with intergenerational deprivation and living in poverty, which are often also subject to various forms of discrimination, are far more likely to have deficiencies in the maturation of their non-cognitive skills. This has important implications for their health, their capacity to learn, whether they graduate from high school, the relationships they form, their later earnings, and the likelihood of adverse encounters with the law.

Intensive interventions in these families early in a child's life can have major beneficial effects, including on nutrition. When nutritional advice is offered to mothers and infants through so-called 'Headstart' programmes, lasting reductions in the risks of obesity are seen. This is clear evidence of the importance of those early years in developing self-control, along with other non-cognitive capabilities associated with healthy behaviours. As every developed country has families in this situation, there is an obvious need to adopt such programmes more extensively. They may seem expensive in the short term but, as Heckman's calculations have shown, they have real economic dividends in the longer term.

The two-legged stool

There is a second reason why the importance of biological development to chronic disease risk has been ignored—namely that a much more simplistic model of gene and environment has been far more comfortable for many scientists and doctors to grasp. Most doctors and medical scientists receive hardly any training in the science of development and there are strong historical reasons in both science and medicine for why development has tended to be ignored. It complicates matters too much for many of us.

Since the Human Genome Project has been completed, the technological capacity to look for genetic variation across our 21,000 genes, any of which might relate to disease, has become a science in its own right. It operates at an industrial scale, devouring enormous amounts of funding and sometimes generating confusing and overstated headlines. But the future offered by this project was projected in a hyperbolic manner even a decade ago. We had the spectacle of Tony Blair and Bill Clinton announcing the unravelling of the human genome to the world—it was certainly an important technological and informatics breakthrough but it is more symbolic than meaningful in its own right.

We heard Nobel laureates making exaggerated claims that they would now find rather embarrassing—namely, that once we had sequenced the genome we would understand essentially everything we needed to know about human destiny. It would be possible, they claimed, to screen populations to determine the risk of disease, then to warn them in time, and to intervene. It would be possible to study the genomic patterns in samples taken from humans with a particular disease, and this might provide information about how the symptoms arose and give us new clues about causation and new treatments. It would be possible to screen the DNA of patients under treatment, to see how their small genomic differences were related to the side effects of the treatments which they experienced. A brave new world for medicine was opening up. Who needed the blurring of focus which developmental biology would add to the picture? It was far too neat and tidy without it.

But as we saw in Chapter 6, the hype and the extravagant claims made at the inception of the Human Genome Project are now dissipating. Hard questions are beginning to be asked. Isn't the possibility of predicting the majority of future cases of chronic diseases, based on the human genome sequence, a mirage? When we get closer, it just disappears. With the wisdom of hindsight we can see that it was always going to be this way—genetic variation is only one leg of a three-legged stool on which our health rests: our development and the way we live form the other two. No stool will stand with only two legs. And it is pointless to ask which leg is most important—

they are interdependent. The two-legged stool gives us no solid basis for understanding variations in risk between individuals and groups, or in looking for opportunities to intervene. There cannot be any firm understanding without including development.

Contributing to this scientific confusion has been a widely held attitude to developmental science which meant that it was left out of the scientific agenda during the early and mid 20th century. Part of the reason was the focus on the genetic basis of inheritance which followed the concept of the gene as the unit of that inheritance, and part of it was the view of many evolutionary biologists that development was irrelevant because it was just a pathway to adulthood—and in their view natural selection only acted on the adult. We now know that both these ideas were wrong.

But there were other reasons for looking askance at development. Part of the reason for dismissing developmental biology followed some well-publicized cases of possible scientific fraud in the first half of the 20th century, which made the subject look very dubious indeed.

Faking it

One of the most controversial biologists of the early 20th century was the Austrian Paul Kammerer, who conducted what even now seems like ground-breaking and fundamental work on development and reproduction in amphibians such as frogs and toads. Working at the privately funded extramural Institute of Experimental Biology (*Vivarium*), Kammerer was convinced that a change in the environment could bring out hidden characteristics in these animals, which could then be passed on to the next generation. In his most famous (and infamous) experiment he induced midwife toads to breed in water by raising its temperature, and he claimed that when this happened the males developed 'nuptial pads' on their feet which enabled them to grasp the slippery females—a feature present in their evolutionary ancestors but not normally seen in modern toads.

Kammerer's finding was dramatic and seemed to support the increasingly unfashionable, and by the 1920s predominantly rejected, theory of the inheritance of acquired characteristics, usually connected with Lamarck. In 1926, it caused bitter scientific controversy and the opposition was led by one of the most famous geneticists of that time, William Bateson—who coined the term 'genetics'. It was then claimed publicly that Kammerer's experiments were fraudulent, a view that was endorsed when it was found that the only surviving toad, albeit one pickled in a jar, had had Indian ink injected into the apparent nuptial pads to make them visible. We do not know whether this was done by a technician to enhance the pads once preserved or whether it was part of a complex fraud. The scientific feud became very personal and very nasty. We may never learn the full truth, as Kammerer committed suicide in September 1926, but recent research indicates that he may have been the victim of a right-wing conspiracy at the University of Vienna against left-wing and especially Jewish scientists.

There were even bigger problems for the status of developmental biology emerging in the Soviet Union. At that time, some of the most important work at the nexus between development and evolution was being undertaken in the relatively young Soviet state where a critical mass of highly innovative thinkers in genetics, evolution, and development had been established. But with Stalin in power, science and politics became confused, and science became subservient to Leninist theory and ideology. Genetic determinism was seen as bourgeois and in conflict with the Marxist belief that the State could mould its citizens to form a new society. Many scientists tried to resist this intrusion of political belief into the process of science, but biological science had become dominated by one man, Trofim Lysenko, who was to have a profound influence on generations of Soviet biology.

Lysenko was an ambitious but poorly trained agricultural biologist who worked on ways to optimize food production. He had come to Stalin's attention because of his claim to have increased production in the collectivized farms. Lysenko's so-called 'science' suited Stalin's politics and, in a rather short time, Stalin was to give him a great deal of control over the Soviet science apparatus. It did not matter that this bogus science had become divorced from reality.

In Stalin's Russia, crop yields were low and this often meant hunger for much of the population, particularly following the failure of the mass collectivization which had led to poor practices. Lysenko was aware of a well-tried and tested procedure called vernalization, by which seeds exposed to cold before they are planted germinate earlier. He wondered if the harsh winters of Russia could be harnessed to condition seeds so that two crops could be planted and harvested each year—what a difference it could make if that were possible! Lysenko's early experiments looked promising, and became dominant in the Russian Academy of Sciences, despite the justified scepticism of its better and more independent scientists.

Lysenko's work attracted the attention of Stalin, who was keen to find ways of optimizing the output of the agricultural sector of the state economy to match the factories of the cities. His science fitted the ideology of the day whereas that of genetics did not—merely breeding new strains of crops took too long and did not yield results as dramatic as those claimed by Lysenko. So Lysenko rose to power in the Soviet system. He aggressively rejected mainstream genetics and biological theory, banishing rivals until he controlled the Russian Academy of Sciences. As time progressed his claims became more exaggerated, going beyond wheat and potatoes to fruit trees and lumber plantations. But Lysenko's work had not gone unnoticed in the West, and shortly after the war delegations of European scientists were dispatched to see it in action for themselves. They couldn't. There was virtually no ongoing work to see and certainly no convincing data published.

It appeared that many of Lysenko's claims that the environment during the earliest phase of plant development could alter growth and improve crop yields were totally false. The scandal broke in 1948 but rumbled on for many months afterwards. With that, Soviet biology lost all credibility in the West and the 'Lysenko affair' became symbolic not only of a widespread distrust of Soviet science, but of the role of the environment in development itself. Tragically, it set Soviet biology back decades and some outstanding work by early Russian evolutionary biologists was essentially lost. Even now, Russian biology suffers from this legacy.

Stories like these are very bad for science. Science requires absolute integrity from those who practise it. Scientists pride themselves on reporting what they have found with great accuracy and even the hint that a researcher is not doing so can be enough to damage their reputation seriously. If there is any question about the scientific probity of an individual, young researchers are advised to have nothing to do with them, that is, they are not to refer to their work and not to engage with them in any way.

Whatever the rights and wrongs of the Kammerer and Lysenko cases, there have been too many examples of unequivocal fraud for any risks to be taken. Unfortunately developmental science seems to have had more than its fair share—perhaps because of its complexity. Recently, for example, the claim by Hwang Woo Suk, a stem cell biologist from South Korea, that he could clone human embryonic stem cells, a technical feat of great importance to the emergent field of stem cell research, caused much excitement when he published his work in the world's leading scientific journal. South Korea started to build a whole industry around him. But all this excitement rapidly turned to justifiable disgust when his work was found to be fraudulent. His reputation was in tatters and he was subject to legal proceedings.

Sadly, there are just too many stories like this, as the stakes in science appear to be getting higher. The commercialization of science, the potential fiscal and career rewards that can now arise from a great breakthrough, drive some scientists to break this code of integrity—after all, science is a human endeavour and some scientists, like other professionals, succumb to temptation. But the code of practice must be protected at all costs if science is to progress and be trusted. The more important the area of research, the more competitive and the greater its implications, the more tempting it is for scientists to step over the line between presenting their ideas in the best possible light and actually fabricating the data.

Scientific fraud is very bad for society too because it slows down progress. But because so many of these cases involved that most difficult of sciences, development, it gained a bad reputation. Scientific opinion leaders turned their attention in other directions.

Splitting up

For much of the 20th century, what makes us what we are was considered in terms of only two processes. One was genetic; the other was the environment. Between them they were considered to hold the keys to whether we are healthy or sick. We were born with a genetic make-up and then had to face the world. For example, if we had the gene that allowed us to absorb the lactose in milk as most people from European stock do, we are likely to have a high dairy intake. If we do not, like most people from Asia, then we have to avoid milk products because they upset our digestion. We term this problem 'lactose intolerance', although in fact the 'natural' evolved state for most humans is to lose the capacity to absorb lactose after weaning. It is only in those descended from some proto-European dairy farmers around 8,000 years ago and some East African dairy farmers around 2,000 years ago who have the genetic mutations that allow them to digest lactose as adults.

Of course no one thought that it was quite this simple when it came to the 'higher' human functions such as behaviour, character formation, and intelligence. It was clear that learning had to play a major role and this really was a developmental process. The way we lived our lives and the environment were acknowledged to play a role, although how much was a matter of opinion. This became structured—fossilized might be a better word—around the nature/nurture debate—one we now know to be very artificial. Are the majority of human attributes largely determined by our genes (i.e. nature), that is by directly heritable processes which could be bred for, in the way that Mendel had been able to do for characteristics in his peas? Or are we born with a 'blank slate', as the 18th-century philosopher Thomas Hume had suggested, upon which early experience and environment (i.e. nurture) could write the story of how we would turn out?

This nature/nurture debate rumbled on, and has had many reincarnations up to the present day, although now most of us realize that it is rather futile. Both processes matter and interact—indeed they are not really separable, as epigenetic biology shows, and do not explain fully what makes us what we are. But as with Lamarckism and Lysenkoism the nature/nurture concept has left its traces in cults and abandoned projects, some of which were influential, costly, and damaging. We need only think of the legacy of eugenic movements, compulsory sterilization, or breeding programmes, spurred on in the mid 20th century by the idealized science of genetics; or the mass testing of children at an early age for IQ advocated by the once famous, and now infamous, psychologist Cyril Burt, based on data on inheritance derived from studies of twins which were found (again!) to be fraudulent after his death. Then, on the nurture side, think of the many nursery and child-rearing fads based on simplistic ideas about environmental stimulation, etc. Despite all our successes, we have not been very smart as a species when it comes to rearing our children.

Apart from the effects on our brain, developmental influences have been traditionally seen as much less important in making us what we are. It came as a surprise to the world of medical science in 1941 when the Australian ophthalmologist Norman Gregg recognized that cataracts and deafness in children could result from mothers having been infected with rubella (German measles) during pregnancy. It conflicted with the current dogma that the fetus was isolated from external influences and it took some years for the significance of this great discovery to be fully appreciated. If the fetus was not immune to outside influences after all, did this mean that fetal development was not as autonomous as previously thought? But these were gross effects which disrupted the developmental programme and caused birth defects such as holes in the heart and disordered bone and brain development, and so were not considered important in the context of human health for the majority of us.

Then in 1961 another Australian scientist, William McBride, showed that the anti-sickness drug thalidomide taken by some women in pregnancy had terrible effects on limb development in the fetus. This was a critical discovery, although McBride's hubris led him later to make unsubstantiated and falsified claims about another drug, debendox, and he ended his career in disgrace—this seems to be a pattern in too many great men of science.

But beyond medicine and within the world of botany and zoology the understanding of the role of the environment in development was growing. Many examples were found in plants, insects, and amphibians where early life events influenced development. The honey bee is a good example. A female larva, hatching from its waxy cell in the hive, may develop into a worker or into a queen. Their destinies will be quite different, like the rags or riches of a fairy story. The worker will slave her life away, collecting pollen and never having any offspring of her own. Meanwhile, the queen languishes in the hive, occupying her time by fighting other queens and preparing for her nuptial flight, when the male drones of the hive will pursue her; successful males will mate with her in mid-air as high as a kilometre above the ground, only to die after this acrobatic feat.

The worker and queen bees share the same genes, yet they could not be more different: the worker bee's mouthparts develop to collect pollen, her metabolism is suited to frequent short flights, and her reproductive organs are shrunken; the queen's mouthparts are suited to fighting, her metabolism is designed for a single long flight, and her ovaries are prepared to lay thousands of eggs. Amazingly, these two very different bees can emerge from identical genetic information. The developmental path that the larva will take depends solely on what it eats in the first few days after hatching—fed on protein-rich royal jelly for only a few days and then with sugary nectar, the larva becomes a worker bee, while prolonged feeding on the royal jelly alone turns the larva into a queen. Interestingly their destiny is not absolutely cast in stone, for if the queen bee dies, some previously sterile female worker bees may start to become reproductively active—their social environment changes their fate. But they never become complete queens—that die is cast soon after the larvae hatch.

We now know a good deal about how two identical sets of genes can be induced to develop into such very different bees as the worker and the queen. If we use agents to block DNA methylation in the larva, it can only develop as a queen. This is the science of epigenetics, which we introduced in Chapter 8. We have seen that epigenetic mechanisms can explain how exposure in early life can have lasting consequences. And we saw that measurement of epigenetic changes at birth can demonstrate a far greater effect of early life on biological consequences than we would have imagined even three years ago. These data provide the basis for explaining the links that the epidemiologists have found between a poor start to life and a much higher risk of developing heart disease or diabetes later in life.

Early markers

Development can no longer be ignored: it is a crucial part of the story of what makes us what we are.

The new insights from epigenetics are compelling. They force those in adult medicine who have ignored the importance of developmental science to think again. Epigenetic markers measurable at or soon after birth could well provide a very good record of the conditions which the fetus experienced in prenatal life. They may be able to tell us how well each baby has responded to the challenges which it met during the nine months when it was effectively hidden from view. Was its nutrition adequate for the growth it was attempting? Was it exposed to levels of hormones which changed the pattern of its development? We think that epigenetic marks will be able to pick up evidence of this with far greater accuracy than just simple measures of weight or shape at birth.

Because these marks are present in every baby, across the entire spectrum of normal growth and development, they can tell us much more. Every baby will have received information from its mother about her life and the world in which she lives—how old she is, whether this is her first baby, what she eats, how much physical activity she undertakes, as well as whether she is fat, putting on too much or too little weight during pregnancy, or developing gestational diabetes. She has taught her baby a very great deal about her world already, preparing it as best she can for the environment in which her baby is likely to live. Epigenetics gives us a way of measuring the impact of all these prenatal lessons at birth.

What can we do with this information? The science is at an early stage and we can only speculate. But potentially it gives us a way of deciding what might be the best diet, lifestyle, exercise level, and so on for each child. Studies are already starting to explore whether we can change mothers' diets in such a way as to get a better epigenetic profile at birth or before weaning. Indeed we might finally have a tool we can use to address a question we really do not yet have the complete answer to—what is the best diet to recommend to a pregnant woman or a prospective father?

Can we use epigenetic information to ask whether a baby might be born with a propensity to lay down fat, or to develop high blood pressure or diabetes? If so, the sooner we help that baby to lead a life that will reduce this risk, the better. This information may help us address the challenge of finding a better strategy to fight the war against obesity and chronic disease. There is an enormous variation in individual risk of disease associated with increased body fat. Some of us may experience a postnatal environment for which our development has not prepared us—perhaps those of us to whom this applies will be those at greatest risk of diseases associated with obesity. On the other hand we know that many of us are equally obese and yet have a low risk—perhaps because our development has prepared us precisely for the world in which we live and allowed us to capitalize on it, to optimize our fat deposition. Epigenetic changes measured early in life provide a way in which we can distinguish between these two extremes, recognizing of course that there is a spectrum in between the two.

In a nutshell, epigenetic processes are involved in making us all different, even if we have very similar inherited genes. So because the risk of disease differs in each of us, establishing our individual risk is likely to involve reading our epigenetic profile.

Several questions immediately arise from these discoveries. The first is whether the epigenetic change actually lies on the causal pathway between early life environment and later risk of disease, or whether it is a signpost along this path, something which indicates a particular state of affairs but is not causally involved. The answer to this important question is not known but, from research in animals and from what we know about the control of the genes involved in conditions such as obesity, it appears increasingly probable that the epigenetic changes are indeed on the causal pathway.

If this turns out to be true then the next question must be—how permanent are these epigenetic changes? Is it possible that they can be reversed, say in early childhood, so reducing risk in an individual? Once again the data from the animal experiments we described in Chapter 8 suggest that this is indeed the case, as administration of some micronutrients such as folic acid or indeed of the satiety hormone leptin can reverse the epigenetic changes in young animals and prevent them developing the phenotype of obesity even if they consume an unbalanced diet as they grow up.

But all this might lead us down a path which we do not wish to follow. Are we really saying that we would propose to give a hormone to young children in order to reduce their risk of later obesity? Well, there are precedents for this in paediatric endocrinology, for example the administration of synthetic growth hormone to children who otherwise would be extremely stunted because of medical conditions, but even that was misused and too many healthy children received growth hormone simply because their parents wanted them to be taller.

We have been at great pains to stress that the relative fatness manifest in many of our young children is an aspect of their normal biological responses, set up in their development. They do not have a disease which we can argue must be treated. Perhaps some generalized intervention might be possible—maybe some nutritional supplement that hypothetically has the same effect as leptin? Perhaps, but we simply do not yet know whether this is possible or safe.

The animal experiments demonstrate that interventions in early life not only reverse the potentially detrimental effects of mismatch or a poor start to life but at the same time reset the epigenetic marks. So this gives us another potential use for such epigenetic measurements, as a possible indicator of the effectiveness of interventions and a monitor of whether they are proceeding according to plan. One source of DNA comes from cells which can be taken from a gentle swabbing of the cheek inside the mouth—we have been able to get ample DNA for our measurements in such a way even from inside the mouths of newborn babies. This is a non-invasive and non-painful procedure and studies taking sequential cheek swabs from babies to examine how their profile changes according to how they are fed are under way in Singapore.

Studying epigenetics at birth and in infants may be the basis for developing a new wave of healthier foods. As epigenetic marks are sensitive to nutrition, we should over time be able to work out which components of what foods lead to better outcomes at different stages of life. While many claims are made about foods promoting health for pregnant mothers and babies, in general these are not supported by robust evidence. Beyond the critical micronutrients such as folic acid, the science is surprisingly hazy. We should be able to do much better using our new epigenetic toolkit, and it is exciting to see that the food industry is starting to take this science on board.

Still no response?

The story seems compelling, but despite this there are many reasons why the importance of development continues to be underplayed both in clinical medicine and in public health. Indeed we feel like the little boy in Hans Christian Andersen's tale who asks, 'Why is the emperor wearing no clothes?' It seems so obvious but we still find ourselves asking the question again and again—'Why is development being ignored?' There are many reasons—some practical, some reflecting vested interests, and some due to just plain ignorance. We have already discussed the history of the basic science and how development came to be largely left out of the modern genomic revolution. Let us now turn to the realpolitik of medicine, public health, and the private sector.

Much of clinical medicine tends to ignore the specialities of obstetrics and paediatrics. After all, these are largely concerned with the normal processes of having babies and helping children through the inevitable problems of early life, aren't they? So in many ways these disciplines are seen as somewhat irrelevant to adult medicine and surgery. Most practitioners in adult medicine are understandably focused on either treating the acute situation or ameliorating the chronic problem and they see no need to look backwards into development. Most problems in adult medicine are dealt with by life-style change, medication, or surgery to treat the symptoms or by various forms of palliative care. It is widely recognized in many developed countries that health services are better equipped to deal with acute situations than with prevention and amelioration of chronic conditions.

And while public health specialists have paid attention to the importance of maternal and child health, the contributions of early life to chronic disease development remain poorly incorporated into their thinking. To some extent the reasons for this narrow view are historical and to some extent they are practical. Throughout its history public health has achieved notable successes, for example in the reduction of infectious illness through better sanitation and vaccination, and the increasingly impressive effects of anti-smoking campaigns especially when these were linked to sales restrictions and excise taxes. These are areas where the division between health and disease is clear and where an agent causing the disease—a bacterium or virus or the tar in smoke, for example—is known. But as we have seen when it comes to obesity, diabetes, and cardiovascular disease the situation is much more complex. The concept of a single causative agent does not work—we cannot live without food and in any event there is enormous variation in how we respond to what we eat. We have spent much of this book explaining why the solution is not as simple as just promoting exercise and diets.

A discipline closely related to public health is that of epidemiology, which is the study of patterns of disease in populations. Large data sets are collected to do this, and cohorts of subjects may be studied for a number of years to look for correlations and associations. For example, it was from such associations that the link between smoking and lung cancer was shown. There is an enormous community of epidemiologists studying cardiovascular disease, diabetes, and obesity, but most of them are researching only adult populations. In such studies it is easy to look at current exposures such as patterns of eating and exercise, but it is virtually impossible to look backwards into the early lives of the subjects. An inevitable bias of such studies is a focus on the importance of what is happening now and an underestimation of or failure to recognize the importance of what happened much earlier in life—where data are not available.

One answer is to study birth cohorts, that is to document babies from birth and see how they grow up, and it was from these data that researchers such as David Barker made the important connection between early life and later disease risk. Such studies are expensive and it takes a long time for the results to become clear. Even designing them is not easy, because it requires being very open-minded. It is difficult or impossible to go back and collect data, let's say on some aspect of pregnancy, at a later date. But now the results of just such studies are emerging in the UK, the USA, Thailand, India, Singapore, New Zealand, and the Scandinavian countries. Very often these studies have been championed by enthusiasts, and often they were not funded by government sources—they were viewed as too speculative, too risky, and too open-ended. Once we start to take a life-course approach to medical research, where will it end? Where indeed.

Drug companies also have a vested interest in focusing on the adult rather than the child, for that is where the greater proportion of income comes from. It is perhaps too cynical to argue that the pharmaceutical industry will not be interested in developing new drugs to prevent chronic disease when they can make a fortune from providing drugs to treat such disease for millions of people for years or decades of their lives. However, if a drug could be developed which would prevent such disease with certainty, following a short course of administration rather akin to an immunization against an infectious disease, then there would be an enormous market for it. But then safety would be a major concern in such an approach; the costs of ensuring that a new drug meets regulatory standards would be high and would take much longer than the patent life of the drug concerned. New regulatory approaches are needed if we are to pursue this route.

In any event the range of drugs licensed for use in children is quite rightly narrower than for adults, and narrower still for pregnant women. We have not forgotten the lesson of thalidomide. So even though in animal studies it is possible to reverse the effects of a poor start to life by drug therapy in the newborn, in reality we are far from prescribing such therapy to children. But perhaps here we are being too simplistic in thinking that a drug will provide the answer to preventing metabolic and cardiovascular disease. Aren't we falling into the trap of looking for the magic bullet again?

A more subtle approach would be to develop a nutritional strategy. After all, unbalanced nutrition across the life-course is in part the cause of the problem, so maybe nutrition can correct the problem if it is introduced early enough. The food companies are starting to see the opportunities here, for example, to improve nutrition of mothers during breastfeeding and to use epigenetic information to improve the composition of infant formula. Here is an example where the food industry can be encouraged to make a difference. It may have little choice in the matter, too, for food is increasingly being recognized as something which has dramatic effects on our lives, and in turn, the regulatory authorities may look to epigenetic tools to assess the biological effects of many food components.

No longer can the multinational food companies stand aloof, and take the view that they will provide a range of foods and nutrients—whether healthy or not—and leave it to individuals to choose what they want. Governments and regulatory bodies such as food standards agencies are now beginning to insist that considerably more information is provided to the public about the content of the foods that they buy, especially packaged and processed foods. Most of us simply don't have the knowledge or the training to make judgements on what to buy and what to avoid.

Increasingly food companies want to address this challenge by developing products which they claim will specifically promote health or reduce the risk of disease. Labelling a tub of margarine as being good for the health of your heart is clearly a great marketing tactic. But how do we know if the claim is true? Indeed one of us found in his local supermarket a packaged food labelled 'enriched with omega-6 fatty acids, proven to improve your heart health'. Really?

Falteringly, regulatory authorities are getting into the act, demanding that the food companies provide evidence for such claims. There is a lot of work to do here for both regulators and companies, and there are differences as to how regulators approach this matter. The foods produced by the global multinational companies may be regulated, but much of the so-called health food supplement industry is not. Standards need to be established and understood. The companies that invest in research-based validation want to be able to distinguish themselves from the multitude of new-age companies claiming health benefits from various food extracts. And the nature of a clinical trial for a drug used to treat a disease is very different from what is needed to develop an argument that a food maintains or improves health. Trials that have disease as their endpoint are just not realistic—they would take 30 years or more to conduct.

Despite all this, some leading companies are willing to take on the challenge and are now engaged in long-term collaborative research with basic and clinical scientists to find firm scientific evidence to support health benefit claims for certain foods. It is easy to see such initiatives as simply a cynical attempt by multinational companies to increase their market share. This, of course, is true to a degree, as the private sector does not normally invest money in something unless it will confer financial advantage in the long term. But there is really no alternative unless we are willing to pay much higher taxes to enable 'independent' organizations, such as government departments or agencies, to undertake the research—and the plain fact is that we are not. We have to keep an eye on the profit motive in the food industry, to make sure that it does not get totally out of control, but surely we all want more clearly labelled and healthier foods to be provided in the same way that we want safer cars, soaps and washing powders that do not cause dermatitis, dyes that are not carcinogenic, and so on. The role of the regulatory bodies in protecting the public is clear and, particularly with foods, the standards must be very high.

As this chapter has demonstrated, there has been a big shift in our understanding of development. Genes and lifestyle alone do not explain what makes us what we are. Development plays a critical role in many ways. Our biology is changed through epigenetics; our behaviour is changed by learning and experience. The more we look at the obesity and chronic disease epidemic the more we see that we have to go beyond 'gluttony and sloth', beyond our current lifestyle and behaviour, and look back to the start of our lives if we are to understand why some of us are more vulnerable to chronic disease than others. And the more we look, the more we understand. There is an enormous change in our thinking under way. Investment in validated approaches early in our lives will likely pay enormous dividends in terms of the pattern of disease in future years.

The problem of non-communicable disease is getting worse—nowhere in the world is its incidence falling—it is rising inexorably in the West and alarmingly quickly in developing countries such as those in sub-Saharan Africa. To imagine that we can simply take failing strategies from Western countries and apply them successfully in the developing world is manifestly wrong. Indeed we need to be certain that what is offered in developing countries is culturally sensitive and appropriate to the populations—they must drive their own agendas assisted by new scientific insights. Further, the growing concern in the West about the developing world cannot be used as an excuse simply for the West to market medicines and health-care services to countries which cannot afford them. We must be sensitive to the economic development agenda that is necessary in such countries, and recognize that a more holistic approach involving areas such as women's empowerment and education, as well as a focus on the beginning of life, will have not only long-term effects on the pattern of disease but also many other benefits.

Such a holistic approach will benefit developed societies too. We know that there is unlikely to be a magic bullet for dealing with the problems of obesity and chronic disease. The reality is that we face the challenge of applying complex interventions to bring about changes at many levels in society—education, nutrition, the food industry, the built environment of home and workplace, etc. We have to learn how to develop for healthy life in a complex world and one which is changing very rapidly. Focusing on our adult or even our adolescent lives alone will not provide the solution—it will come too late for most of us.

11

From Words to Action

There are many factors which create barriers to an effective strategy for winning the war on obesity, diabetes, and cardiovascular disease. We have seen that merely focusing on adult lifestyle will inevitably have rather disappointing effects when looked at in terms of a whole population. For some it will help a lot but for many it will only slow their progress down the path to illness. We have seen that there is enormous variation in how some people get fat and suffer chronic disease in the modern world while others appear more resistant. We have seen that there is enormous cultural and societal variation in attitudes to food and why healthy lifestyles and the motivation to stay healthy are, for many, hard to sustain. We have learnt that development matters in many ways—both through changes in our biological make-up and through what we learn when we are young. We have seen that our biology is influenced for life by the behaviour of our parents and possibly our grandparents, by our life as an embryo and as a fetus, and then by how we are fed in the first few crucial years of life.

There is still a lot to learn but we may have the tools now to answer some of the critical questions, such as: what is the best way of feeding babies from the time they are conceived? We have reviewed the exciting research of the last few years which has shown how important epigenetic and developmental processes are in explaining why we get fat and why some of us get chronic disease. Surely we can now use that information to start doing something rather than just talking about the problem? Indeed it could be argued that with the knowledge we have now it would be unethical to wait any longer. But as we have seen, there is already a large investment in the current approach which focuses on the adult, and the blinkers are still firmly in place. While it would seem obvious to look elsewhere when the current strategy is failing, few have been ready to admit that the war will be lost if we do not adopt some innovative and new approach. We have enough knowledge and it is time to do so. So where do we start?

Warming to the cause

An analogy with global warming may be apposite. Climate change is another kind of environmental challenge affecting the human condition that is also to a large extent of our own making. The first thing that was necessary before we could deal with the issue was to set out the scientific basis for action and then to establish an attitude change—at both governmental and individual levels. The science is complex—it involves multiple feedback loops and very non-linear systems in which not everything can be or is known. Yet decisions have to be made because the consequences of waiting could be horrific. And the science cannot be fully separated from people's values and beliefs.

Much of the public debate over whether man-made climate change is real or not is artificial, a substitute for a real debate over how to respond to the problem. The real issue is one of intergenerational equity—whether to take actions now that have a cost for this generation in order to help the next, or to wait. Waiting is based on the hope that, even if the problem will be worse if left untouched, a technological solution may present itself, just as it has done in so many other situations which have challenged humans. Rather than debate about differences in values, the issue underlying much of the motivation of the so-called 'sceptic' movement, the discussion is reframed around complex science and the extent to which man-made climate change is occurring. Very few unbiased climate scientists think that this question needs much debate—there is more to find out, certainly, but the role of human activity in driving global warming is accepted by nearly all those who do not have vested interests in refuting it. At long last, policy makers have accepted that this consensus merits a discussion about action.

The analogy between obesity, chronic diseases, and climate change can be drawn in several ways. The science is certainly very complex, it has multiple dimensions, and there are many things we still do not understand. There are vested interests in operation too, which would prefer to retain the status quo. And it is also a matter of values—how much emphasis to put on the health of the next generation and how much on the lifestyle of the current one.

In the climate change arena two approaches have been adopted to reconcile these conflicting views—mitigation and adaptation. Mitigation is about incentives to reduce greenhouse gas emission, through either fiscal incentives or green technologies. Adaptation concerns the active search for technologies that will allow us to cope with a much warmer world at some time in the future, even if we cannot prevent such warming. The technologies for adaptation that have been discussed include massive geo-engineering projects, literally on a global scale.

We would equally argue for a two-pronged approach to obesity and the chronic diseases. On the one hand, we must continue the current efforts aimed at promoting healthy living—mitigation—but in doing so we must understand their limitations. On the other hand, we must start thinking much more seriously about new solutions for the next generation—adaptation.

Shifting gear

Any action plan will require a shift in resource, both fiscal and political. Lip service to the importance of the early stages of life is easy. It is like saying education is important—no one can seriously disagree with such a statement. But many societies do not value teachers highly or pay them well, and some have not made universal education compulsory. But then we will meet the very valid argument that resources are not limitless—so, as in any aspect of public policy, we have to be more specific as to how they should be deployed.

And this is where good science is so important in informing the policy makers about their options. A focus on promoting optimal development is no different from the anti-smoking campaign. We did not wait 30 years to find out with absolute certainty that reducing smoking would lower the incidence of heart disease or lung cancer in the population. The science was already good enough— from animal experiments that carcinogens in tobacco smoke caused cancer, epidemiological studies of the links between 'pack years' of smoking and disease, and so on. The problem for a long time was the uncertainty about this scientific data which was deliberately spread by the tobacco industry. But when that battle was finally won, governments moved fast. Legislation followed, doctors and teachers stopped smoking, advertising and vending machines were banned, taxes on cigarettes were increased, smoking was banned in public places, etc.

The recent introduction of immunization against the papilloma virus, which causes cervical cancer in women, followed a similar course. Once the scientific link had been made between the viral infection and cancer, and the vaccine had been developed and tested, it became feasible to vaccinate pre-pubertal girls safely and on a large scale. The introduction of this vaccine was far less controversial than might have been predicted by sceptics. In general, society did not feel the need to get caught up in the seemingly enormous barriers of explaining to these girls 'You have not reached puberty yet but after you do you might have unprotected sex with a range of partners who are also sleeping around a lot. We are not saying that you will behave like this, but if you do your risk of this nasty form of cancer will be higher. So, to be on the safe side, we're giving you this injection.' Instead of being mired in a complex debate about modern sexual mores, governments understood the reality of the risk, accepted it, and, took action.

The evidence is now clear that early development is an important piece of the puzzle that makes us what we are, and we need to use that information in formulating more effective strategies to improve the human condition on a global basis. The science is increasingly robust and is very consistent. It screams 'Development matters!' The developmental dimension explains why some people are more and others less sensitive to getting obese. It turns out to be a story that affects every one of us and not just those who are born small or prematurely—we are all creatures of our genes, of the world we live in, and of the way we developed. This new science offers exciting possibilities. It explains more of the biology of disease than previous attempts and it will allow us to measure early markers of disease risk and to explore possible interventions and monitor them. And it is more than just epigenetics, because we now have many other tools to look at development afresh. For example, with new imaging techniques we can look at body fat developing in different parts of the body, from birth throughout childhood. While there is much more to learn about this new dimension, the science of development is now sufficiently robust to demand action.

Because there have been a number of dedicated scientists and health professionals looking through the developmental lens for years, much of the work to formulate the best approach already exists but it is not being implemented systematically. While there may be differences in emphasis on what to do in different countries and different societies, there is a common set of themes.

Masterly inactivity

Almost a decade ago a technical committee set up by the World Health Organization spent days debating the most appropriate types of interventions. It comprised over 30 experts from both developed and developing countries. They applied themselves diligently to the problem, and their work was followed by consultation meetings in several developing regions across the globe. One of the authors chaired this committee and both of us were involved in the subsequent consultation. Tellingly, the experts had initially been asked to focus on measures to reduce the number of babies of low birth weight, defined as those weighing less than 2,500 g, throughout the world. But even before the work started, the scientists charged with organizing the meeting realised that they had to shift the focus away from such a narrow perspective and aim the discussion at giving all children the best possible start in life.

One of the benefits of such expert groups is that it enables scientists of different perspectives to look at the problem from several angles. There was a considerable variety of disciplines and countries involved—high-technology and low-technology approaches, nutrition, women's health, paediatrics, epidemiology, and basic science. World Health Organization reports go through multiple cycles of feedback and debate before they see the light of day publicly and individual bias nearly always gets subsumed into a consensus. So such reports ought to carry considerable weight.

The report of this group was unequivocal in its conclusion that the global burden of early and later life disability as a result of impaired fetal development is huge, both in developing and in developed countries, and that the promotion of better fetal and infant development would enhance social and economic health and well-being in many populations. The benefits it listed included school performance and skills, health during adolescence and adult life, better physical work capacity and greater learning skills, increased productivity and economic gains, a reduced burden of infectious diseases, and, central to our argument, obesity, diabetes, and cardiovascular disease.

The report identified many opportunities for population-based intervention, using a public health approach, and others that would be more appropriate on an individual basis. All of the report's recommendations applied equally to developed and developing countries, although their relative importance, it was recognized, would differ. None of the recommendations will come by now as a surprise to the reader of this book—and none really should have surprised public health professionals worldwide at the time.

Before life starts

Much of the report focused on the condition of the mother before she became pregnant. It was clear that women needed to be in a much better nutritional condition when they conceived. It was pointed out that far too many women in the world have their first child at a very young age—strong sociological forces lead to this being the case in many societies. But this means that young girls do not receive an adequate education and are disempowered. Biologically it is clear that optimal fetal development is more likely if at least four years have passed from the time a girl has her first period and when she conceives. Only then has her pelvis reached a maximum size, which allows the fetus to grow optimally, and only then has her biology reached the point where she no longer needs to hold back nutrients for her own growth at the expense of her fetus. In much of the developing world this is not the case. Strong recommendations were made to encourage a delay in first pregnancy. This would have greatly empowered women in many societies by allowing them to stay longer in education—or indeed to receive an education at all. There is now growing evidence that the empowerment of women is a key step in the economic advancement of every country and the importance of allowing every girl a chance to delay reproduction until an appropriate age must not be overlooked.

Given what we now suspect, we would probably want to add in the health and nutrition of the father as well. Indeed, in some trials in South Asia it has been found that unless such interventions also include the father, the mother will still miss out because she will be seen as subservient to him; even if a food supplement is given to her, it will be reserved for the father.

Staying the course

Other recommendations of the World Health Organization report focused on the woman once she became pregnant. These included specific recommendations about adequate and balanced nutrition and weight gain in pregnancy and efforts to support the mother during pregnancy through reduced physical workload and stress. Many women in the world walk miles each day to collect water and undertake heavy, physical farming work even during late pregnancy, and often pregnant women do not have priority in the family when food is limited. Far too many women are subjected to physical abuse during pregnancy, and the resulting stress hormone changes can affect the baby.

The need to reduce smoking in pregnancy was affirmed by the World Health Organization committee, and alcohol and drug exposure remains an ongoing concern. Malaria and HIV-AIDS are major problems during pregnancy for far too many people—malaria in particular invades the blood-rich placenta and the parasites consume the oxygen and food that should go to the fetus. Malaria is a major cause of fetal growth retardation in developing countries and the importance of continued efforts at its eradication is obvious.

Born and fed

Other recommendations of the committee focused on the birth process itself and then on the baby once born. They emphasized that many babies are still born without a trained midwife. If the delivery goes badly and the mother dies or becomes infected, the baby will inevitably have a bad start to life. This is an ongoing issue, and in the last year we have seen much attention, especially from the Gates Foundation, on improving the conditions of birth. Several hundred thousand women still die each year in pregnancy or childbirth—clearly, addressing this is a priority in its own right but we should also recognize the long-term costs of poor obstetrical care.

Lastly, the committee focused on the importance of exclusive breastfeeding for several months. But then, and since, little attention has been paid to post-weaning foods. The committee concluded that much more attention should be given to individuals in terms of matching postnatal nutrition to the circumstances into which they had been born.

While the recommendations above were framed for the developing world it is easy to see how they can be extended to the developed world. They were published six years ago and yet have had little impact. The report remains on the shelf. Why were agencies and governments unwilling to take steps to implement such recommendations?

On the shelf

As usual in politics, there are several reasons for this lack of action. Of course it takes more than the report of one World Health Organization committee to change the emphasis of healthcare recommendations, so we should not expect too much. But the report never even progressed through the World Health Organization machinery itself. Part of the explanation may have been political. The report gave high prominence to the rights of girls, to their empowerment, and to delaying the age of first pregnancy. Maybe it was this that buried it. After all, this was the era of the Bush administration in the USA and contraception was considered by some on the political far right to be equivalent to abortion. Further, there were many patriarchal societies in

Africa and Asia where this kind of argument would fall on deaf ears. But change has to start somewhere, and where countries in the developing world have empowered women the evidence of economic and social progress is clear.

Other reasons for the report not progressing very far are more pragmatic. The division of the World Health Organization dealing with it was small and not well linked to the big agendas of the time—such as HIV-AIDS. And with personnel changes the momentum was lost. When the report was finally made public, along with those of some of the regional consultation committees, it seems not to have been discussed further within the World Health Organization to any significant degree—it does not get a mention in subsequent reports, such as those dealing with chronic disease. But perhaps its influence grew slowly within the organization. The current Director General of the World Health Organization, Margaret Chan, spoke in 2011 with passion about the need for young women to be educated, of their empowerment, and of the importance of breastfeeding and a healthy environment for the first two years of life after conception for every child.

It was clear then, as now perhaps, that even the influential governments of the developed world have few scientific and medical advisers who really understand the issues. Why should they? They are highly intelligent and well-educated people, but even if they are medically trained they will not have spent much time during their studies, or since, considering the long-term consequences of the developmental environment. Development forms only a very small part of the syllabus for doctors in training. The long-term consequences of poor development are only now beginning to be clearly seen. So are we expecting the experts to advise their governments to take a new course of action? We are.

We have turned more than once to the analogy of global warming. The long-term consequences of the epidemic of obesity and chronic disease are calculated to be of the same magnitude as those of global warming, at least in economic, health, and social terms. Just as with climate change, these problems require recognition of the science of what is seen as a 'new', but is really a rather old, field. In the developing world their solution will necessitate coming to international agreements on courses of action, and in the developed world as well as the developing world this will require a cross-party approach because addressing the problems will take longer than two or three electoral cycles. But in the end the actions have to take place at a local level, and this means having the political will to implement them in the face of possible opposition from competing interests. Greenhouse gas emissions will not be reduced in the UK, for example, unless we can resolve the issues of coal-burning power stations, petrol- and diesel-powered cars and trucks, and the cost of insulating our houses. The government has to engage with the energy industry, with the car and transport industries, and with the building trade. They know the issues, they can see the solutions . . . but they hesitate.

No appetite for it

Awareness is one thing but action is another. If there are behavioural and nutritional aspects to achieving a good start to life, then everyone in a population needs to have enough understanding to make healthy choices. Sadly the quality of nutritional information and nutritional education is generally poor in most countries. Yet the evidence exists that even nutritional education starting in preschool can have considerable long-term benefits. We need educators trained both in nutritional science and in the pedagogy of how to engage children of various ages in the subject, as the approach needed differs greatly between preschool and teenage years. We need a coherent lifelong approach to nutritional education—the Japanese already have such a remarkably effective approach. And that education must be made available to both parents and children. Family eating and food purchase habits can be changed—children are important determinants of what a family eats.

But all this will be meaningless unless there is a more consistent and intelligible method of food labelling to explain its contents. This has been surprisingly controversial, but even well-educated people cannot convert a kilojoule to a calorie, and very often they understand the meaning of the latter but not the former—even though they are measures the same thing, i.e. the energy content of food. Portion sizes are equally confusing, and energy per 100 g means little. In the array of largely meaningless micronutrient ingredients, so often listed as a percentage of recommended daily allowance—who understands what that really means?—the simple information we want to know is lost. In an effort to achieve simplicity, some countries have gone to the other extreme by introducing traffic light labelling systems on food. This does not really help either because we all have a clear idea of what traffic lights mean, and they do not relate to food. Does green mean you can eat as much as you want and red that you should stop eating any of this food? Not really.

And the dieting industry does not help—rather it confuses. Of course dieting products are not really aimed at keeping people healthy, but at the cosmetic market. It thrives off its failures. The biology of weight loss is gradually being understood. It is now clear that in the same way as some people put on weight while others are less sensitive to an obesogenic environment, the ability to lose weight and then to keep the weight off differs markedly between individuals. In general, diet and exercise will lead to beneficial weight loss but it is now apparent that most people will drift back to their set point established by earlier weight gain. It may take a few years but the tendency to return to the unhealthy state will be there—the hormonal and brain drive to eat to the higher set point remains operative for many people. It can be overcome by drugs but most weight loss drugs have side effects. That leaves bariatric surgery, with its own side effects, as the ultimate solution. Not a great choice.

And if we shift our attention from fat to diabetes and heart disease the picture is not very different. By the time we come to the attention of the physician it is generally too late to do anything but to treat the disease medically. In some cases weight loss will reverse the high blood pressure or reduce the insulin resistance, and certainly exercise and healthy eating are essential parts of treatment, but again, prevention would be better, and in the end, much cheaper. We believe that we are being realistic rather than negative in saying this—we have pointed to many ways in which a difference could be made, albeit over a generation.

As we focus on nutrition we must engage better with the food industry and the supermarket chains from which we buy the majority of our food. So we are asking our governments to engage again with some of the economic giants—with their acknowledged entrenched interests—to see if new accords can be reached. Burgers and fries may not be healthy but vast profits can be made from high volume sales of them at a low cost to the customer. They are cheap and convenient, and—there is no point in being sanctimonious about this—anyone who has looked after small children on a rainy Sunday afternoon in a city knows that it can be easier to keep them quiet by giving them this junk food. This should just be a rare treat rather than a staple, that's all. We cannot avoid the chemical reality that fat is energy dense but at the same time contains the flavours that make food enjoyable. And junk food is tasty—humans have evolved to have a taste for foods that help to build up body fat, which are generally sweet or salty.

There are always profits to be made from new technologies. The rate of investment in start-up companies in 'green-tech' and in sustainability is a direct outcome of both governments and the private sector recognizing the new realities of climate change and environmental degradation. The environmentally aware consumer may be willing to pay substantial sums to adjust to this new world. We are beginning to see similar trends in the food industry. This industry has long recognized that health claims allow a premium to be placed on the product, so it is not necessary to reduce the profit margin as sales increase, as is common with other foods. This is most clearly seen with foods made for babies and infants, where the prices charged for simple but safe and clean foods are higher than the ingredients would normally warrant.

But quality control matters—we have seen the tragedy in China, when such control was poor and children were fed milk contaminated with poisonous melamine that unscrupulous farmers and middlemen had added to increase profits. And baby foods should not replace breastfeeding, ideally for six months after birth, but the potential for nutritional supplements to mothers while pregnant or lactating and for better post-weaning foods is obvious. Companies are starting to make research investments in this direction. They should be encouraged, provided that the research is rigorous and any claims made about their health benefits are well evaluated.

All parents want the best for their children, and health-promoting foods seem an obvious market. This market is still perceived as small compared to that of the needs of adults for fast, tasty food, but it will become larger as the economic powerhouses of India and China continue to develop. Indeed they are regions of the greatest need, as health costs are beyond the means of the majority of those who need medical care—so now is the time to act.

The longer view

Just as with global warming, the issue of promoting a healthy start to life requires taking a longer-term view. Governments are not good at this. A policy to promote health in the population which will not be particularly evident for another generation is not likely to attract votes if an opposition party can offer a tax cut next month. Long-term interventions do not deliver results in the time frame of an electoral cycle, and they also commit the government to long-term resource allocation. But having said this, we should remember that governments already do this—after all, that is the logic behind state-funded education. It seems to us that we are not thinking clearly enough about the need to invest now for a highly productive next generation in other ways too.

And, at last, some governments are beginning to see this. The UK independent review on obesity by the Foresight group, commissioned by the Department of Health, was published in late 2007. It is a complex document, containing scenarios for possible intervention at various levels in the obesity epidemic—in education, by reviewing the role of industry, through implementation by legislation, and so on. It includes diagrams of Byzantine complexity that look like the innards of a supercomputer and are guaranteed to deter the casual reader. But its conclusions are clear. To quote.

> Of 17 different potential governmental policy responses across built, health, fiscal, research, educational, regulatory, social structure and family domains, the only one with a significant impact on obesity in all three scenario contexts explored was to promote/implement a programme of early interventions at birth or in infancy.

Let us hope that this report will not languish on shelves in Whitehall as others have done at the World Health Organization. But as we have seen, there are many reasons why this outcome is a real possibility.

Don't blame us

Throughout this book we have been very conscious and concerned about the concept of blame. The naive belief that being fat or developing diabetes or cardiovascular disease is simply a reflection of voluntary lifestyle choices is widespread among the public, many public health officials, and politicians. So blame can easily be attached to 'gluttonous and slothful' overweight individuals. This is not a trivial matter—and indeed one powerful weapon in campaigns to reduce smoking is the stigmatization of the smoker. But we must not stigmatize the obese, particularly the morbidly obese. This is because much of the supposed by blameworthy activity may not be under their voluntary control, or at least may not be easy to control. There are powerful biological drivers that make weight loss very difficult to achieve and to sustain. Secondly, stigmatization creates stress, and this itself can lead to greater weight gain as rising stress hormone levels can induce both more eating and greater fat deposition.

But the blame issue runs much deeper. It impacts on political ideology and policy. If it's 'all your own fault', why should the State remedy it for you? Many from the more libertarian part of the political spectrum would take the view that the State should not have a role in matters of personal choice. That is why political parties in countries like New Zealand and the United Kingdom have found it difficult to venture too far towards trying to control what people eat.

The blame game is extended to the food industry, which is sometimes vilified indiscriminately for its part in the obesity epidemic, and for having nothing but the profit motive on its agenda, regardless of the cost to human health. No doubt there need to be tight controls on what the industry markets and how it advertises its wares. Most of us like to feel, however, that we can choose what to eat, so portion size control and clear labelling are needed to help us consider the consequences of our choice. But from what we can see, much of the food industry is willing to move in this direction—after all, it basically wants to keep selling food and will not be slow to pick up a change in public demand and taste.

The cynics will say that the food industry will go with its customers some way down this path, saying the right things to reassure them about its best intentions, but only so far. Some of the leaders of public health, such as Margaret Chan of the World Health Organization, now argue that we have to test the industry's resolve here—to offer to engage with them in a joint initiative to promote health and wealth across the world. If they do not step up to the plate (in more senses than one) they will only have themselves to blame. This is a better use of the blame tactic.

Parents are no longer able to provide the necessary knowledge to the next generation about healthy eating. Thus, we contend that the State has a greater responsibility than is generally recognized. There is no doubt that the focus on blame has inhibited progress—it is easier to blame the individual than to tackle the problem. And in our work we have become very concerned about how to focus on promoting healthy development without giving parents a sense of guilt. We know that this is a real challenge—it frequently crops up in questions in the public lectures which we give. 'Oh, so it's all our fault is it?' parents exclaim, often with some anger. This is wrong because we are dealing with the normal processes of plasticity—it would be the equivalent of saying you should blame your parents for teaching you your first language.

We evolved to have our biology influenced by that of our parents—unlike some animals that hardly have parent-offspring relationships. Just as it is inevitable that you will learn to speak their language if you live with them as a child, it is not their fault if you are the first-born or if you were born smaller because your mother is only 155 cm tall. In Japan is it women's fault that they have reduced their weight gain in pregnancy? No, it is driven by societal attitudes to body shape and misleading advice from their obstetricians. We need to get beyond this superficial approach, which can be dangerous. We cannot allow this new biology to be interpreted in such a way as to give parents—and women in particular—a sense of guilt. If we do, new scientific advances will be overlooked and future generations will not reap the benefit of what we now know.

In any event, is it anyone's fault that they live in the modern energy-dense world, surrounded by fast food and sedentary leisure pursuits? Our biology is designed to make the most of it, even if it does have the unintended effect of inducing obesity and increased disease risk.

Ethical issues

The new research we have described is opening up exciting possibilities, but also new ethical dilemmas. We already know from our work with children that specific epigenetic changes at birth predict the level of body fat and the degree of vascular injury nine years later. And a large body of experimental data in animals confirms that this biology is important. Further factors which are known to play a role in influencing the risk for the child, such as maternal smoking, obesity, age, diet, and whether a child is first-born or not all influence these epigenetic changes. The power of this technique is manifest from the sheer strength of the association. For some specific parts of the epigenetic profile, the preliminary data suggest that measurements at birth which tell us about the prenatal experience—including the effect of the mother's diet in pregnancy—can account for a considerable proportion of the variation in fatness in the children many years later. Not only are the amounts of fat that we are talking about large—differences of several kilograms of fat between children—but the predictive nature of the epigenetic mark is stronger than any purely genetic effect and explains more of the influence on a child's body composition than anything else ever reported.

The ethical issues arising from these observations cannot be ignored. They are similar to the concerns that emerged when genetic diagnosis first appeared on the horizon. There was considerable concern that genetic information would become the basis for setting the premium for an individual's life insurance, for example, and laws were put in place to protect our genetic privacy. To a certain extent the broader ethical issues have emerged more slowly than anticipated because genetic prediction turned out not to be as informative as its early protagonists had hoped. In some situations, such as the diagnosis of parents carrying single gene defects which cause diseases including cystic fibrosis and Tay-Sachs disease in their child, genetic diagnosis has still not achieved its goals. There are many doctors in the world who believe that there is great potential for better genetic screening, particularly for certain forms of childhood cancer. Sometimes these are more common in certain populations. This used to be termed an ethnic link, but now the term 'ancestral' is preferred for such markers. Even so, the implications have not been resolved— individuals in some populations are very sensitive about their ancestry, especially if there are tribal, religious, or other cultural implications. So the widespread use of neonatal blood samples is debated. These samples are routinely used to screen for treatable metabolic diseases such as phenylketonuria, and are usually stored for a period of time—and can therefore be valuable for research.

In the light of the issues raised by genetic screening, the future of epigenetic measurements is still not clear. Optimistically, we think it may be useful at an individual level in ascertaining the level of risk and thus suggesting how best to manage the future. It may help us to monitor interventions aimed at reducing risk and to optimize approaches to improving the start to life. But we emphasize that we are talking about risk and vulnerability—a person's epigenetic state determines in part how they will respond to the environment. Early interventions can change those responses if they are instituted in time. If we know a baby is likely to be on a higher risk pathway for chronic disease, we would recommend prolonged breastfeeding and attention to diet and exercise to reduce that risk. Perhaps research will find even more effective interventions in the near future, which can be made more culturally and individually specific. In addition, an effective use of epigenetic information will provide new knowledge about how best to optimize conditions before the next generation is born.

When we move from Western culture to other cultures, we are on even more shaky ground in dissecting out rights and the ethical issues. But we can point out how this knowledge can assist in reducing the burden of the economic and nutritional transitions. Take, for example, the age of a woman at the birth of her first child. We discussed earlier the problems of teenage pregnancy. In many parts of the developing world girls are married very soon after they start their monthly periods—in some places even before this time—and they become pregnant soon after puberty is complete. This problem is made worse by the fact that in many societies married women are expected to undertake a substantial amount of physical labour even during pregnancy: working in the fields, carrying water and fire-wood, etc. Often they are the last to eat in the family, after the husband and children. From what we discussed, we can envisage the signals which the mother will be sending to her developing fetus. This is a mismatch scenario in the making.

Learning in time

Resolving this problem, of course, comes down to the education and empowerment of women, but this is not a panacea and it has to be handled with great sensitivity. In particular, solving the problem must also involve the education of young men. In some societies girls who have started to menstruate are at particular risk of being raped if they are not married, and once devalued in this way they are less likely to be married. They can drift into prostitution or other forms of service which will not ensure a good future for them or their children. So to a certain extent, the young-bride scenario confers some protection on girls. However, once married they may be expected to work in the home or to become mothers. If they were attending school they are likely to stop doing so. This limits their ability to take control of their lives and to develop their own careers and it also severely limits oppor-tunities to explain to them what they should do in relation to their health and that of future generations.

One of the obvious approaches to resolving the teenage pregnancy problem is to ensure wide access to contraception, but this is not acceptable in many cultures. Moreover, in some cultures anything which might be viewed as a Western imperialist influence is likely to be resented, and this will be counter-productive. We saw something similar play out in the tragic delay in accepting the use of antiretroviral drugs to treat the South African HIV-AIDS epidemic during Thabo Mbeki's presidency.

Even in the absence of well-organized educational structures in developing countries, all need not be lost in the drive for the empowerment of young girls. We should not underestimate the influence which social contacts with peers can have in influencing behaviour. For example, a pioneering study by Anthony Costello and colleagues from London was able to show that good birthing practices could be advertised and organized through social networking. Given that Costello and his team were working in rural Nepal, we don't mean Facebook or Twitter—we simply mean discussions around the local well and at the market. Women are far more likely to adopt a behaviour if they hear about it from a friend or relative whom they respect than if they are simply told it by a health worker or see it on a poster. We all tend to trust information received from neighbours, relatives, and friends—whether over the fence, in the pub, or at the workplace—more than from some government-sponsored initiative which seems to smack of interference in our lives.

What we are discussing here is referred to as 'health literacy' and there has been considerable research in this area over recent years. It shows that the progression towards such literacy goes through phases where we assimilate information on health issues, turn it over in our minds, internalize it, and then begin to use it in a critical way to decide on courses of behaviour, actions, etc. It is only perhaps at this later stage that we start to communicate our conclusions and give recommendations to our family and friends. Perhaps surprisingly, the research shows that even relatively young children are good at this activity and that they can very often become crucial influences on lifestyle and health issues within the family. This was certainly what was found in Southampton when the impact of children's attitudes and preferences on the diets of families was studied, but it extends far more widely to include a huge range of aspects of life. Children naturally represent the future, and they begin to take control of this future, as well as of their own lives, at an earlier age than is perhaps often recognized.

Paying for it

If in the developing world girls are conceiving too early in their reproductive lives, in the developed world there is a problem at the other end of reproductive life too. In the UK the average age of first pregnancy is now 31 years. Because this is an average, clearly many women are conceiving much later than this. Evidence is accumulating that the signals sent by the mother to her fetus change if she is older, potentially creating a greater mismatch, and there is concern that this may contribute to the rising risk of diabetes and/or heart disease later. Once again this is an issue that will have to be tackled on a wider cultural scale.

One achievement of second-wave feminism was to liberate women from the close link between their sexual lives and reproduction; to give them the opportunity to plan when they have children in relation to their careers, their choice of partners, and so on. Women face a difficult choice with regard to important career moves which might mean that they must remain in full-time employment or undertake further training at a time when they may also wish to be starting a family. No society has managed to make this choice easy. Feminists would argue that until reproduction itself is adequately reimbursed financially as an activity, the choice between career and family will remain an agonizing one for many women and their partners. Some of those who believe that the obesity problem lies largely in adult lifestyles would even argue that the careers of women have taken them out of the kitchen, reducing the time that they might have had to cook traditional meals and giving them the cash to buy faster options that are less healthy.

Even though no society has tackled the issue of reproduction as a wage-earning activity head on, many developed countries nonetheless attempt to mitigate the situation by providing financial support during late pregnancy and nursing. The problem then arises of the level at which this support should be set and for how long. In most developed countries child support terminates when the youngest child enters school, but in a few it extends until the child leaves secondary school—the value of this prolonged support is highly debated. In some countries such as New Zealand it has been suggested that this support makes it better financially for a young woman living in a disadvantaged situation to have children than to take on a job. This is very controversial but there is enough anecdotal information to suggest it may influence some teenage girls who have dropped out of school, and so we can see that a well-intentioned strategy to resolve one problem might make another one worse.

The UK's coalition government and its opposition are currently engaging in discussion on the importance of these issues and their impact on families. For example, it has been argued that the provision of child benefit allowances should now be limited to those who pass a means test and have a low income. This is perhaps basically fair, but it is tricky because however the rules are set, there will be some who unfairly miss out and others who can exploit the system. Such problems can be addressed but they raise deeper issues. Should couples be discouraged from having more children than they can afford to support, even without the allowance?

Who will decide the answers to these questions, and in whose interest should the considerations be made? Throughout the developing world it has been found repeatedly that poverty is associated with larger family size. There is no surprise here—especially in some societies where it is the tradition for the children to remain in close contact with their parents, and in fact to support them as soon as they are able to do so. This is particularly true of rural agricultural communities in the developing world, just as it was true of Britain in the Middle Ages, because children provide the next generation's labour for tasks such as agricultural work. But as prosperity improves, so family size shrinks.

Economists such as Jeffrey Sachs would argue that saving the planet through reducing population growth is intimately linked to economic growth. It would appear that families have fewer children both as their economic prosperity grows and as child survival becomes more reliable. And yet this too creates a paradox for, as we have seen in both China and Europe, the development of fat and the risk of later obesity and perhaps diabetes or cardiovascular disease are greater in a first-born child. We need a demographic shift, in that we need population growth to slow down if we are to sustain our increasingly resource-constrained world, but we also need to pay attention to the quality of life of the next generation. It is clear that the pattern of heart disease and diabetes is different in different countries. Particularly in countries that have undergone rapid recent nutritional transition, it occurs at earlier ages than in the West. We need to confront this challenge if the drivers to reduce family size are to be sustained.

Drag forces

There are enormous institutional and structural impediments to progress and the issues we have just raised illustrate the complexities. But beyond that is the problem of inertia in both the scientific and medical communities. Finding ways to promote a healthy start to life does not have the instant appeal of cancer or HIV research, perhaps because prevention grabs fewer headlines than cure. Governments have short-term objectives linked to the electoral cycle, informed by treasuries that adopt an econometric approach.

International agencies such as the World Health Organization also suffer from inertia and are often very encumbered by protocol—they can spend longer debating whether a representative from a particular country should be at a meeting than planning a strategy on which the lives of thousands depend. For the World Health Organization, the issue is also complex because its members are the 192 countries which it represents, not representatives from civil society groups such as the World Diabetes Foundation, or indeed from the private sector. This situation is changing, as it must if we are to make any real progress in the prevention of chronic disease, especially in developing countries. In some areas, such as infectious disease, the World Health Organization has played a superb role, but sadly, in the area of development it has been a different story up until now.

In low-income countries the role of voluntary philanthropic agencies such as the, Gates Foundation has thus become dominant, if only because they have far more funding to disperse. Donors are entitled to define where and how they want to spend their money, and Bill and Melinda Gates and Warren Buffett represent enormously generous donors. However, their funding is often targeted at specific, relatively short-term goals, for understandable reasons: this is where results can be seen very quickly, rather than the more difficult holistic approach which is necessary to tackle longer-term problems, such as improving human development and reducing the risk of chronic disease. However, the dependency of many developing societies on philanthropy skews the locus of control and the health promotion agenda of governments.

Lastly, and perhaps strangest of all at first sight, is the problem that arises from too much enthusiasm. Whether we look at attempts to promote physical activity in school children in developed societies, or at those offering nutritional support in developing countries, we find that there is a plethora of organizations avidly taking on the task. Some may be sponsored by government departments, some by international agencies, some by global philanthropic organization, and others by local charities.

In reality there are just too many cooks in the kitchen and very often they have different recipes and approaches, so they can waste time and resources by duplicating efforts and not jointly building the infrastructure needed for a sustained campaign. Sometimes they may even compete—a phenomenon which has been seen on a more dramatic scale when several agencies are involved in relief operations in famine or earthquake situations. We desperately need global coordination here, to bring these organizations together. We could then not only pool the resources which they have at their command but also deploy them according to their particular skills and personnel base. More and more we see the need for an international legal system to deal with issues such as genocide or torture. These are issues of human rights, and surely the right to the best possible start in life should be placed on an equivalent level internationally. It may be that empowering—and appropriately funding—an existing organization such as the World Health Organization would meet this need. We don't know. But surely leaving something that is so fundamental to human life to take its chance in a haphazard way among the priorities of a range of disparate organizations is irresponsible, if not downright immoral.

12

A Call to Action

Ignoring the messenger

At the end of this book, we have a simple message for governments, agencies, and aid organizations. The current approach to obesity, cardiovascular disease, and diabetes is not working. There are multiple reasons and we have discussed some of them. They lie partly in the fundamental nature of the problem: we now inhabit an obesogenic world which we have not evolved to live in healthily; the development of the problem has been fast—like an epidemic— and insidious, so that by the time it emerges in a society it is too late to prevent it; cultural and individual motivational issues have been ignored; but, most importantly, the science suggests that a key part of the story has been overlooked. It is no longer possible to ignore new discoveries in developmental biology. The time has come to look again at why we are losing the war against obesity and chronic disease, and to choose some strategies that are likely to be more effective.

We know that many people across the globe are not in a healthy place in their lives, but moving them to a better place is not easy and may not work at all for some individuals. To a great extent this is because we have been asking the wrong question. Instead of asking what we have to do to make these people healthy, we should be asking how they arrived at this point, what path they took to travel to this unhealthy place. It is as if we have arrived at the scene of a crime and are now trying to figure out how to stop it, rather than looking for clues to the events leading up to it. But the fact is that we have arrived too late. We have forgotten about human development and how the processes operating in our early lives will shape our future, literally the shape and size of the fat in our bodies. Just because we are struggling to help those who suffer from obesity and disease risk as adults, let's not forget the need to prevent this problem recurring in the next generation.

We have presented the case that a fresh look is needed in the war against obesity, cardiovascular disease, and diabetes. Winning the war clearly involves more than just increasing our worries about how fat we are and much more than accusing each other of gluttony and sloth. We have reviewed the science and the biases and blinkered views that have affected the way strategies have been chosen in this war. We have argued for a much more holistic approach, one that recognizes the cultural, social, individual, community, and developmental factors in play. Just because it is complex does not make it impossible to address. We cannot afford—literally—to wait and let a large fraction of the world become unwell and disabled. But it is all very well sounding this call to action. What action are we proposing?

First, there needs to be a far better engagement between scientists and the public. How that engagement should be conducted is a book in itself, but we can make a start. We have seen the conflation of values and ideology which has allowed science to get tangled up in the blame game that places responsibility almost entirely on individuals. That this is not correct could be explained clearly. It is difficult to motivate people if they do not own the problem—in no small part that contributes to the magnitude of the failure of current efforts. And people are not likely to own the problem if they do not understand clearly what it is.

True, the science of human development is complex and there are many things that we do not know. But this should not be an excuse for not communicating it. Any new ideas in science can engender fears and here we are dealing with something pretty fundamental: what makes us what we are? what explains why some of us do well and some poorly in this modern world? The scientists engaged in this area have a duty to explain the ideas, and their implications, clearly to us all. Most scientific research is funded by the public in one way or another. It has authority in a modern democracy only to the extent that it is understood and accepted. Too many scientists forget this or just do not understand that such communication is part of their job.

How might we apply these new scientific insights? The potential for prediction in early life of those at risk of later disease using a combination of epigenetics, genetics, and measurement of other risk factors is a good starting point. To be able to predict which children are more at risk of developing diabetes or cardiovascular disease is a good thing if prevention at that stage is possible, but it also brings problems. Do we want our children to be labelled? What possible discrimination might this lead to, for example from insurance companies or employers? Answers to these questions will depend on a conscious effort by scientists to communicate early and clearly the benefits of new technology and not to shy away from the ethical and practical issues that arise. Failure to do so will leave the wider public, and politicians too, confused about the issues—as the furore over genetically modified foods or stem cell therapy demonstrated. A Luddite approach cannot work—whether we like it or not, seeking new knowledge is fundamental to humans and new knowledge will lead to new technological applications. Post-genomic, that is epigenetic, science is a key part of the next biological revolution. It could improve the quality of life for many—if it is properly applied.

We should not allow ourselves to be daunted by the fact that we are dealing with a complex problem. We have stressed that a single intervention does not fit all scenarios, just as the simple remedy of reducing energy intake and increasing exercise has had limited success in adults. It is always easier to arrive at a viewpoint or to devise a slogan that conveys a simple and direct approach but, as always, the devil is in the detail. There is no single magic bullet. The biology is complex and we should exploit this fact by recognizing that a multidimensional approach is needed. While we encourage healthy lifestyles we can still work to optimize the developmental factors which determine how pathogenic any particular lifestyle is.

Many public health campaigns focus on reducing the number of people at the extreme of a range—perhaps those who are clearly ill. Yet from a health perspective, and in terms of saving money in the long term, it is more important to shift the health of the majority of the population—of those of us who are 'normal', even though we may be at lesser risk—in a favourable direction. That said, this does not mean spending the same amounts of money on improving the health of all of us. Some sections of the population, especially the poor and poorly educated, will require more investment to shift their health to a more favourable position.

Next we need to do better at championing health and nutritional literacy. The more we understand about our bodies the more able we are to make better choices. Most of us believe that the role of the State is to empower its citizens to make healthy choices rather than to tell them to do so. This requires that the State take the lead in ensuring a level of health literacy and nutritional education from the earliest ages. Too much has changed to expect knowledge to percolate through families—active education is needed.

The more we understand about healthy eating from an early age, the more likely we are to eat better throughout our lives. Much of this book has focused on the earliest stages of life, and the more we learn about development the more we realize the importance of the period around conception. But a large percentage of women do not plan their pregnancies. And even if they do, the information available about what they should eat is very basic and unattractive. Ensuring the best start for the next generation requires that potential mothers—and probably fathers too—eat more healthily throughout their reproductive years. Such a change in habits requires an understanding of the implications of intergenerational health.

Not such a bad idea

One argument sometimes put forward is that, while these suggestions seem like a great idea, we would have to wait a generation to find out whether they work, and the world cannot afford to invest in such a speculative manner. This is a false argument on both direct and indirect grounds. The use of epigenetics and other biomarkers will likely enable us to show short-term benefit. For example, we can now use rather simple and non-invasive measures to study how the body develops in infants or when blood vessels start malfunctioning.

But even more obvious is that these initiatives will do a lot of good in their own right, in the short term as well as in the long term. Empowered and educated young women will play a much greater role in social and economic development in their communities. The measures we recommend will in themselves reduce the number of premature births, neonatal deaths, and cases of infant illness, and will also improve brain development in children. Each of these justifies the suggested approaches in their own right.

So the argument for waiting for even more research to be undertaken is simply prevarication. The real argument relates to intergenerational equity. Those who argue that our limited resources for health should be focused solely on adults alive today are failing to recognize the right to health of the next generation.

251

Ally or enemy

We need to find a way to make the food industry an ally, not an enemy. It made sense to vilify the tobacco industry, but it is illogical to extrapolate from that strategy to the food industry. We have to eat; we do not have to smoke. We must address the bad practices of the food industry—the marketing of junk food to children, the ridiculously large portions served in fast food outlets. But let us be realistic because, for much of the world, food security—that is, a reliable and safe food supply—is the bigger and more urgent issue. A flourishing food industry, active at every level in every community, is essential if food security is to be sustained.

Some futurologists argue that a failure of food security is potentially a grave risk to world stability and will be the source of future conflict. Somehow we need to engage the food industry and give them incentives to make products that meet their goals while serving each population's needs better. Such a dialogue is now on the cards, even at the World Health Organization, in an attempt to build a multi-stakeholder approach to solving the problem. If the food industry lets us down by concentrating only on the short-term profits which serve their immediate vested interests, then more serious controls and constraints will have to be put in place. But provided that they are honest and transparent about where their conflicts of interest lie, we have to work with them.

Innovative approaches are emerging but they require lateral thinking and collaboration between groups that may previously have been at loggerheads. In an earlier chapter we described how gestational diabetes confers the risk of chronic disease on the next generation. Recently we visited some colleagues in China who were well aware of the issue. With support from the food industry and the Chinese Ministry of Health, Tony Duan at Tongji University in Shanghai and Huixia Yang from Beijing have established over 100 centres to provide nutritional advice to young couples and trained 150 health workers to give that advice. In a period of less than two years over 170,000 people had attended these centres. A key focus has been to manage dietary intakes during pregnancy to avoid excessive fetal fat deposition—and they believe that they are succeeding.

We know that many paediatricians in the West believe that it is unacceptable to collaborate with the food industry, particularly in the area of infant foods, under any circumstances, just as virtually all scientists would agree that no collaboration with the tobacco industry is ethical. There are many memories of the active discouragement of breastfeeding by infant food companies when they promoted their formulas in developing countries in the 1970s—well-meaning parents shifted from breast to bottle with devastating increases in mortality from infection in their children. A lot has been learnt from that experience by the infant food companies and by doctors and regulators. It is time to move on. We have to accept that the very organizations which have been part of the problem must also be part of the solution.

Don't throw the baby out with the bathwater

While this book is focused on the role of development, we would not want the reader to interpret what we have written as saying that nothing we can do in adulthood is of any value. Of course there is much we can do to be healthy adults. What we are saying is that it is hard to make sufficient changes in adult life to bring individuals back onto a low-risk pathway for non-communicable disease. Some of us will benefit from weight loss programmes but many will revert in time to where we started. Clearly, diets low in saturated fats, sugars, and salt are of value for those on the high-risk pathway to chronic disease, and exercise both improves insulin sensitivity and adjusts the body's energy balance favourably. But the reality is that at a global scale a focus on these measures alone is not working. We cannot rerun the early life development of millions of people around the world to reverse the steps they took many years ago. Adult interventions are too little, too late for them.

This is not to say that some current programmes should be discontinued. Among all the adult interventions there can be no doubt that the campaign against smoking has been highly successful and has had major effects in reducing the risk of cardiovascular disease, lung disease, and lung cancer. There have been major advances in many countries in reducing smoking through a mixture of strategies—social marginalization of the smoker, legislation to restrict where they can smoke, vilification of the tobacco industry, and taxation to increase the price of tobacco products. We need to keep reinforcing these approaches.

It remains a tough battle. One of the best ways to reduce cigarette smoking is to stop advertising. This has been achieved on television in many countries. Another way to do so is to insist that cigarettes are sold in plain packages. The Australian government is trying to do this but the tobacco lobby is rich and aggressive. The tobacco industry is even threatening to reduce the price of cigarettes if the government carries through their plan.

And what should we do about a country such as Malawi, where the economy is almost entirely dependent on tobacco growing? There is plenty of water in Lake Malawi which could be used to irrigate other crops, but is the international community prepared to provide the assistance that Malawi would need to switch from tobacco growing?

Creating coalitions for battle

When we are fighting a war on many fronts, and losing, it can be a good strategy to combine forces to achieve greater penetration on a smaller number of fronts. This is exactly what is needed in the fight against chronic disease. We need to integrate our approach to the problem across the life-course, from conception to maturity and middle age, by making it part of education, primary care, welfare, women's and children's support, and so on. The list is not short, but each of these domains currently operates with its own bureaucracy and its own goals and priorities. If we are to make real progress we will have to join up these activities. Not only will this make success more likely, and probably save money too, but it will ensure sustainability.

After all, one of the critical differences between the 'epidemic' of non-communicable disease and other truer epidemics of infectious disease is that the problem will not be solved all in one go. An epidemic of a new strain of swine flu can be stopped in its tracks—permanently—by developing the appropriate vaccine and using it effectively to prevent new cases occurring. We are safe then, until the next epidemic strain appears. But with diabetes and cardiovascular disease we will have to keep up our endeavours to hold them at bay for generations to come, no matter how effective we are in reducing them right now. That is, unless some genius invents a time-machine which will allow us to rerun our evolution so that we remain naturally healthy in an obesogenic world. Or unless we all wake up tomorrow and decide that we don't want to live sedentary lives in warm accommodation and have easy access to tasty food . . . neither of these possibilities seems very likely.

When we turn to the developing world, the need for a more unified approach to chronic disease prevention becomes even more obvious. We know that the problem will not be fixed quickly because, unlike in the developed world, it is only just beginning. We have not yet seen its full impact in this generation and the one immediately following, let alone come to grips with what will be needed to keep such disease at a reduced level. On an international scale the large organizations such as the World Health Organization, which should be able to take a long-term view, have relatively little funding to invest. More and more health interventions depend on the contributions of large philanthropic organizations such as the Bill and Melinda Gates Foundation. Regrettably, however, these large philanthropic organizations have not yet really engaged with the challenge of chronic disease prevention, even though they are strongly committed to reducing infectious disease, reducing poverty, and promoting socio-economic improvement.

Why is this? It is not through lack of information, because several representations have been made to such organizations at the highest level by influential scientists and doctors. We think that the reason for this lack of response comes from the very nature of philanthropic organizations. To a large extent they are driven by the vision and the desires of a small number of individuals, very often the wealthy individuals who established the organization or their initial scientific advisers. At least in the first instance such people—and this is no discredit to them whatsoever—naturally want to make a difference and to see the effects of the funding they provide in a relatively short period of time. Moreover, and particularly in times of financial duress, they are cautious about becoming involved in schemes which might have to run for many years in order to produce a sustained difference.

The lessons learnt in the 20th century from food aid programmes in the developing world are still fresh in many people's minds. The answer to starvation is not simply to provide food—not unless we are ready and willing to provide it for an indefinite time. Sooner or later we will have to stop, and know that we leave behind a problem unsolved as we walk away. Replacing food aid with sustainable agricultural and light industry schemes was the answer, in the hope that populations could become self-sufficient. For diabetes and cardiovascular disease it may be even more difficult and we are only just beginning to see what the longer-term sustainable solutions might be.

So it is easy to see why organizations such as the Gates Foundation have focused on infectious disease prevention. If they can send a team of health workers into a part of the world such as rural India and vaccinate young children against polio with a few drops of vaccine on the tongue at the cost of only a few dollars each, then we can see how attractive such a scheme might be. One can divide the total amount in dollars that one is willing to spend by the cost per child of vaccination and come up with a figure of the number of lives saved—of people who will not get polio, ever, during their life. If one does the calculations right, it may even be possible to eradicate the disease entirely in the region, and thus deal with the sustainability issue as well. After all, this is what has been achieved for smallpox in many developed countries.

Infectious disease prevention is an extremely worthy venture and one which we should not belittle, and we can see why it might take priority over investing the same amount of funding in a long-term campaign to prevent chronic disease, for example, by educating young girls in the same part of rural India. We can't simply move in and set up a school and educate children for a year or two and then get back into our vans or helicopters and leave, as we could for a vaccination programme. Education is a long-term business and nothing much will be achieved from a short-term programme that cannot be sustained.

The Gates Foundation spends so much on prevention of maternal and infant mortality—which is linked to Millennium Goals 4 and 5—and it is but a small extension of that magnificent effort to also invest in those same mothers and infants for the longer term. Surely this makes sense and would build on their contributions to date. We know enough to see specific actions that could make a difference— keeping girls in school, nutritional education and support for women and infants, promoting family planning: these are simple measures that could make a real difference.

There is another dimension to this issue too. In comparison to government-funded bodies, philanthropic organizations are relatively unaccountable. They take advice from experts, whom they choose independently, and evaluate the success or otherwise of the programmes which they fund in their own particular ways. We can see why they do this—it's their money after all—but it risks giving a bias to the work. The charity or philanthropic organization may have a board of trustees to satisfy and a scientific advisory board which it must convince, but otherwise it operates in a relative vacuum. This is the traditional way in which philanthropy has operated for well over 100 years, but given the influence which charities now have over international bodies, we need a new form of more aligned strategic planning involving both agencies and the donors.

The blame game goes global

There is general agreement that we need integrated action at the global level, although there may be disagreement about the shape of that action. As the epidemics of obesity and chronic disease take hold and spiral out of control in countries like India and China while continuing unabated in the West, we see grave risks ahead. Many developing countries will simply not be able to handle the burden of disease and we will have the nightmare scenario of economic development leading to rising expectations at the very time when the productive section of the population becomes unwell. This will damage development and have global consequences. And beyond that there is the risk that these countries will blame the West for their ill health. It results, they might argue, from the Western-controlled multinational companies encouraging them to adopt more Western lifestyles for financial reasons. The geopolitical consequences could be very unfortunate.

By the time this book is published the United Nations General Assembly will have held a special high-level summit for world leaders to address the issue of non-communicable disease, with particular emphasis on the developing world. This is only the second time since its formation that the United Nations has convened a summit to address a specific health issue—the previous summit addressed HIV-AIDS. It has been informative to watch the build-up for this summit. Different countries and interest groups came to it with very different motives and agendas. There were those for which this represented an opportunity to sell high-technology medicines and health systems to developing countries. Some of the companies manufacturing these have been pilloried in the past for not providing such treatments and systems at low cost to developing countries. Now they can envisage improving their reputation while still retaining a profitable business, if inexpensive generic drugs or equipment can be developed in conjunction with government and philanthropic support, to be sold in vast quantities in the developing world. As with the food industry, there is nothing inherently wrong in this, but the potential conflict of interest has to be recognized.

Other groups lobbying the delegates of the United Nations summit were those for which this was an opportunity to ram home the 'gluttony and sloth' message and to continue aggressively with the failing blame-the-individual agenda of the West. Some of these groups wanted to use the opportunity to attack the food industry; others wanted to focus on specific interventions or solutions, following the anti-smoking model. Some, again with good reason, argued that many chronic diseases such as cancer have their origins in infection, and so approaches similar to that used successfully to prevent infectious disease should be the priority. And there were representations from faith groups, from ethnic minorities, and from other civil society organizations, all of whose voices had to be heard. Incorporating the views of all these disparate groups into some coherent and achievable action plan was an unenviable challenge.

The World Health Organization took responsibility for coordinating the delivery of whatever plan was drawn up at the summit, although in reality, of course, it had been decided to a large extent beforehand. The World Health Organization had to grapple with this by involving a large range of organizations in the preliminary discussions. But when we wrote this in May 2011, time was very short. It was disappointing to see how dominant the World Health Organization itself had been in this initiative, with the manifestation of its own internal politics, to the exclusion of other agencies in the build-up to the meeting. We believe that a much more integrated approach was needed, involving many agencies, from the UN Development Programme, UNESCO, and UNICEF to the UN Women programme and the Food and Agriculture Organization. And beyond the United Nations there are many other agencies that have an important role to play, such as Christian Aid, Save the Children, Médecins sans Frontières, Oxfam, and so on. And then there are the big foundations: Gates, Ford, and Rockefeller; the big charities such as the Wellcome Trust; and the private sector. We can only hope that the World Health Organization is up to this challenge.

It seems to us that the problem is of sufficient magnitude for a new agency of the UN to be needed—there are perhaps too many vested interests operating now for one to get a coherent view. And however the UN takes the lead, it must do so informed by science rather than by politics.

Our leaders may decide that the issues are too complex and too intractable and that the political fallout from addressing them will be too great. They may be deterred by the cost of the action needed now on a global scale, despite the argument that the investment will pay off enormously in the future. They may conclude that we need much more research—which is true enough, but only if it is directed towards evaluation of action.

The kind of science upon which action should be based is sometimes called 'post-normal' science. This is science which is complex and where there are, and will remain, many uncertainties. Such science cannot be fully separated from issues of societal values and attitudes. Yet the matters involved are urgent and action is needed. Climate change is an example of such science, as is food security, as well as infectious and non-communicable disease. The philosopher of science Heather Douglas in her recent book *Science, Policy, and the Value-Free Ideal* points out that in such situations the first question has to be whether there is enough evidence of sufficient quality to act, while acknowledging that this evidence will not be complete. Even more importantly, there may be errors in the available evidence. The question then boils down to the risk of doing harm from acting prematurely on the basis of evidence which turned out to be flawed, versus the risk of doing nothing when the available evidence indicated that action should be taken. This can be a tough decision.

In this book we are arguing for action—focused on mothers and children—to reduce the risks of non-communicable disease in large sections of many populations. Our arguments are based on a growing base of knowledge and evidence. So what does the 'post-normal' approach tell us? Are the risks of acting on incomplete or flawed evidence too great? If we are wrong, we will have promoted women's and girls' empowerment and women's and children's health, and this can only have positive effects on national and personal development. The costs of such interventions are not great. It is difficult to see *any* risks in taking this course of action. On the other hand, if we accept the argument that the focus of intervention should remain on the adult, and do nothing to promote a healthy start to life until we have substantially more information, we will place the next generation at greater risk of chronic disease and potentially incur an enormous cost. We rest our case. With what we now know, it is clear that the balance of arguments weighs heavily in favour of action. We can put it off no longer.

13

Seeing and Believing: The Fat Emperor Has No Clothes

Down and dirty

Ignaz Semmelweis was a young physician working in the 1840s in a charity maternity hospital serving the under-privileged women of Vienna. But 'serving' might be the wrong word, for this hospital was actually a place of death. Alarmingly, one in ten women admitted to a particular ward to give birth in the hospital would die. The cause was a severe fever, starting soon after childbirth, called puerperal fever—'puerperal' being the Latin word for child-birth. It is now known to be a form of blood poisoning due to bacteria entering wounds and tears in the vagina and cervix during delivery. But in the mid 19th century this mechanism was still to be discovered.

It was general knowledge in Vienna that being admitted to this ward was a death sentence, and women begged to be sent to have their babies in another ward at the same hospital where, strangely, the risk of death was much lower. Some women said that they would rather deliver on the street than in the deadly ward—the risk of death from delivering on the street was indeed less.

Semmelweis, at 29, was at an early stage in his career and his superiors would maintain that he still had much to learn. But he could not ignore this problem. He became obsessed with finding out why this one ward had such a high rate of maternal death while another was much safer. There was nothing obvious: the two wards used the same approaches to managing the childbirth and the mothers after birth; they used the same equipment and protocols. He looked into every possible detail of what could explain the horrific difference in outcomes. One ward was more crowded than the other, but the overcrowded ward was actually the safer one, because that was where women preferred to be. The only other difference which he could see was that the first ward was used to train medical students and the second ward to train midwifes, but that seemed trivial and irrelevant. Surely that alone could not explain the difference . . .

Semmelweis pondered and pondered. Then in 1847 a medical colleague who was a close friend died from a fever, after being accidentally pricked by a student's scalpel while they were jointly performing a post-mortem. The post-mortem findings on his friend looked to Semmelweis very similar to those of the dead women from the less safe delivery ward. Although the 'germ theory' of disease, which would later explain the transmission of illness from one person to another, was not yet known, Semmelweis wondered if some toxic particles from the dead body being examined had been passed on by the scalpel to the body of his friend, leading to his death. If so, could the same particles from the corpses be transferred from doctors' and students' hands to women in labour or after delivery, and cause their puerperal fever?

Suddenly, and sickeningly, Semmelweis realized the possible significance of this idea. Medical students did post-mortems as part of their training; midwifery students did not. Suppose the students went straight from the post-mortem room to the maternity ward—if their hands carried the dangerous particles, perhaps they could pass these on to the women in labour and give them blood poisoning. Was the problem due to nothing more complicated than the medical students having dirtier hands than the midwifery students? It was a testable hypothesis: Semmelweis insisted that medical students and doctors on his ward washed their hands in a chlorine solution after they did a post-mortem and before examining a woman on the ward. And their instruments were also to be washed. He chose chlorine as his washing solution because it got rid of the smell of the rotten flesh from the post-mortem and he guessed it might therefore be destroying the unknown deadly particles—he was not to know that chlorine is a powerful disinfectant, the active ingredient of household bleach today.

Within six months of introducing this policy onto the ward where the medical students trained, the mortality of women dropped dramatically—it even fell below that of the ward where the midwives trained. In some months no women at all died on the ward. It was a dramatic change and it was clear to Semmelweis that hand washing in chlorine solved the problem. Surely this evidence would be accepted by everyone? He started to publicize the idea. He wrote letters to other hospitals, describing his life-saving results, and they were soon published in the major medical journals of that time. But were his ideas of hand and instrument washing adopted? Not really, not in many places.

Instead Semmelweis came under intense attack from his colleagues and superiors. His theory did not fit with the orthodox models of disease favoured at that time—that illness results from changes in the balance of 'humours' in the body. He could offer no sensible scientific explanation for what he had observed—only repeat that he had seen the results to be dramatic. The principle that direct observation should outweigh prejudice and dogma was not yet well accepted in science—maybe it still isn't (think of climate change denial). Other experts thought that there was nothing original in what he was saying—another stock criticism of a new idea. Anyway, it was insulting to the medical profession to suggest that they should have to wash their hands—how could such gentlemen be unclean?

Then politics intervened, for Vienna was very unstable at that time. Semmelweis was forced out of his job and he moved to Budapest. Undeterred, he again introduced his chlorine hand washing rule into the hospital—again with the same dramatic results, and again the local medical establishment ignored him and railed against adoption of the procedure. Finally the pressure took its toll, and Semmelweis was admitted to a mental hospital. He died soon after admission, at the age of 47—ironically from fever which was probably caused by an infection following a beating by the hospital orderlies.

It was only some 20 years later—after the discovery of the role of germs in causing disease by Louis Pasteur in Paris—that the importance of Semmelweis' brilliant insight would be recognized. He had produced a paradigm shift in medical practice that has undeniably saved millions of lives. It is a tragedy that he did not live to witness this shift.

Ignoring the evidence

The story of Semmelweis has some parallels with the one we have told in this book. When there is a problem, and the strategy to solve it is not working, we need to look at the situation afresh, at what might really be going on, and get beyond established dogmas. We need to look at the empirical data and observations, rather than basing our actions on belief and fashion. We have to take our blinkers off. The answer may then be surprisingly obvious.

There are many other examples in medical history where cutting-edge science has been ignored or considered implausible—sometimes at great cost to human life. Earlier we described how Mont Liggins discovered in 1972 that steroid hormones given to mothers in premature labour prevented their babies dying from lung disease. But it took another 20 years for the USA to adopt steroid therapy as standard and all sorts of excuses were used to ignore Liggins' data. Might the acceptance have been faster if he had made the discovery in the USA rather than in New Zealand? We don't know. But all too often, in medicine as in other areas of life, there are vested interests that consciously or unconsciously influence the strategies adopted.

More recently we have seen the denial of the role that the human immunodeficiency virus plays in the origin of AIDS, which effectively prevented the use of antiretroviral drugs in South Africa. Many lives were lost because Thabo Mbeki's government refused to accept the overwhelming scientific evidence—albeit from research in developed countries—that a virus was involved. Diverting arguments were used and ineffective remedies were promoted instead. In other places we have seen authoritative claims that condoms do not help stop the spread of HIV-AIDS, despite the overwhelming evidence that they do, simply because the use of condoms does not fit with the values of one particular religion—and at what cost? It can be very difficult for new scientific discoveries to overcome preconceptions and dogmas when the evidence conflicts with values, be those values professional, political, cultural, or economic.

Large scientific, medical, pharmaceutical, and public health enterprises have been built on the presumption that the current paradigms of how to manage the burden of obesity, diabetes, and cardiovascular disease *must* be right. Cynically we might say that private sector organizations, such as the pharmaceutical or the weight loss industries, have invested far too much in this strategy to allow new ideas to change it. But apart from the money, there is considerable investment in ego, reputation, and the careers of many scientists, doctors, public health practitioners, and agencies, and this is not helping. There are many reasons why it may be easier to ignore the fact that we are losing the war.

But the facts are undeniable: the incidence of obesity and the number of deaths from non-communicable disease are continuing to rise in the high-income countries, although the mix is changing because of the major beneficial effect of a reduction in smoking. And we have seen how the incidence of diabetes and cardiovascular disease is exploding in developing societies. Most of the strategies we are now using in the West, other than those against smoking, are clearly not working—can we expect them to work more effectively in developing countries? We are sceptical.

Whose fault is it?

The life-saving achievement of Semmelweis resulted from his developing a strategy based on evidence rather than dogma. His evidence was not sufficient to change the minds of his colleagues, at least during his lifetime, partly because it inevitably attributed a certain amount of 'blame' to a causative agent—the medical students who did not wash their hands. His medical colleagues had other and very deeply rooted ideas about the causation and the blame—unbalanced 'humours' in the patient herself. We see some parallels between this story and the one we have told in this book. Are we challenging dogmas about where the blame lies for diabetes and cardiovascular disease?

Most of the strategies to address the epidemic of obesity, diabetes, and cardiovascular disease in developed countries have been based on the assumption that the primary problem is behavioural—deal with smoking, persuade adults to consume fewer calories, particularly less fat and salt, and to exercise more, and all will be well. This lifestyle-focused approach also fits in with Western libertarian philosophies which seek to maintain the individual's liberty to choose, and reduces the onus on the State to intervene. But unlike smoking, people have to eat, and there is an argument that the State has no business to interfere in our lives in this respect. Indeed many governments have found to their political cost that there is an electoral price to pay for over-interference in individual choice.

Besides, the simplistic view is that, unlike smoking, there is no 'passive' obesity, and so the State does not have to intervene to protect the innocent third party. But this is wrong: there are indeed many ways in which obesity and chronic disease can be transmitted passively from one person to another—both by social transmission and biologically across the generations.

It has become clear that it is intellectually dishonest to base the global approach to non-communicable disease prevention on the assumption that voluntary lifestyle choices are the primary cause of the problem. We have seen the many ways in which cultural, social, and physiological factors conspire to place most individuals in a situation where it is almost inevitable that they will become obese or develop diabetes and cardiovascular disease. The key issue is that we are all exposed to lifestyles that put us at risk and for many of us our capacity to make the changes essential for safety are limited or impossible because of what has happened to us earlier in the life-course. Where the cultural and social factors prevail, they are not easy to overcome—partly because they too can become hard-wired and irreversible through early life. The biological arguments are compelling.

Having said this, we would not want the reader to come away with the idea that there is no health value in eating better and exercising regularly (and certainly smoking should be actively discouraged). Far from it, for where this can be achieved it will have real benefit—anything that improves the match between our biology and our life-style promotes health and reduces the risk of disease. But these strategies largely apply to Western countries, and at best can only ameliorate the problem. Transferring them to the emerging countries will be difficult—except in the case of smoking reduction where some developing countries are starting to make real gains. But it is not realistic to imagine that we can effectively reduce the incidence of diabetes and heart disease simply through lifestyle improvement in emerging countries using similar strategies to those that we have been using in the West. Far deeper issues are involved that need to be addressed.

Even if these behaviour changes were effective, they would have limited impact. Most people in the least developed world do not place as much emphasis on future events as those in the West. Surveys in developing countries have shown that, while all parents want the best for their children, people in difficult circumstances are also realists—what happens today and tomorrow is far more important than what *might* happen in 20 years' time. This is essentially the point that Dan Nettle was making in his evolutionary argument, that people in poor circumstances live their lives at a faster pace. Effective lifestyle intervention will also be of limited effect until there is more equitable economic and social development, both within and across societies.

The simple fact is that through our technologies applied to modern industrial agriculture and food processing, and through the built environment, we have created a world that provides energy and nutrients in proportions beyond the capacity of our bodies to cope. This failure of our bodies to cope is most obvious in the increase in visceral obesity and the insidious onset of diabetes and cardiovascular disease, processes that start much earlier in the life-course than most experts realize, and often before we are born.

But while we may be able to change our nutritional world to some extent through healthier foods, better diets, and exercise, it is totally unrealistic to imagine that we can return to some historical world. The world has more than ten times the population of 200 years ago, and ensuring that no one starves must take priority over worries about chronic disease. Moreover the totalitarian nature of the policies that would be needed to exert the necessary levels of control on the food industry would be unacceptable in virtually every society. We cannot deal as societies with more acutely harmful practices and agents, so is it realistic to imagine that we will be able to do so with food? Ideas about food and its social value are central to every culture, every religion, and every society. And many cultures have different perspectives on the ideal body image too.

There are certainly unacceptable and undesirable practices within the food industry which must be tackled urgently. The aggressive marketing of high-energy, nutritionally poor foods to children must be stopped. There is no value in alco-pops or high-energy caffeine-loaded 'power' drinks, all of which can have adverse health consequences. There is a growing industry of health foods sold at a high premium where in most cases there is no evidence for the claims made, and well-intentioned people are having their pockets emptied by the marketeer. Perhaps financial disincentives can deal with very unhealthy foods, but care will be needed to ensure that the disadvantaged do not become more disadvantaged through food insecurity. And is it not paternalistic to say that the answer lies in controlling what poor people can eat rather than in dealing with the fundamental question of why they are in that situation?

But we also have to defend some aspects of the food industry. We cannot stigmatize it in the universal way which we could the tobacco industry. Rather the world needs the food industry to be engaged constructively in the enormous challenge of food security, arguably the most direct challenge to most developing nations, which will get worse as populations expand and the planet continues to warm.

If food is to be an effective weapon in our global war against non-communicable disease, we need to shift the focus from claims about the 'new age' health foods to developing scientific evidence on which to base claims for 'foods for health'. There is little doubt that nutrition and nutriceuticals will be an important part of the solution to the problems of diabetes and heart disease, but claims for health benefits from particular foods should be scientifically regulated and based on evidence, so that we can make informed choices. The regulatory mechanisms in place for food and health claims are not well developed, are confusing, and inhibit rather than encourage research. This should be a priority for regulatory agencies around the world. We need to create frameworks within which the food industry can work with the health sector to produce products that genuinely do help and which justify the research investment by companies.

But in the end the food industry both creates the market and also changes the market in response to consumers' preferences—that is the fundamental nature of the free market economy which most societies espouse to some degree. And that creates another challenge for us—to educate consumers about what they should buy and what they should eat, not just for this generation but for the next. And that will not be possible without consistent, easy-to-understand food labelling that is designed to help rather than confuse.

It is often said that it is only junk food that poor people can afford to buy. That is often the case but it need not be so—in many cases it is the lack of nutritional awareness that leads to many of us making poor choices. Nutritional education for people of all ages must be a core part of our strategy in both high- and low-income countries. It is obvious to us that this must be a starting point, but it requires coherent and well-informed educators provided with context-appropriate support materials. Nutritional and health literacy is as important as any other form of literacy for a healthy world.

And in the developing world much needs to be done. For example, the tragedy of the heavy subsidy of corn by the US government cannot be underestimated. It was started by Earl Butz, agricultural secretary in the Reagan administration, but it continues today. It drastically changed the nature of the processed food industry and the type of fats and sugars used in the food supply across the world. It is depressing that domestic politics in the USA makes this subsidy, which has global impact, untouchable even though the First Lady, Michelle Obama, has proclaimed her ambition to tackle childhood obesity. The removal of these distorting agricultural subsidies, and those operative in the European Union, would have considerable impact. Opening up the international food trade would greatly assist the economies of many developing countries, for which agricultural production and export to the West remain the most rapid way for economic advancement. But sadly the West still uses tariffs and domestic subsidies to inhibit the developing world's capacity to sell their food globally.

Development squared

The paradigm shift which Semmelweis brought about resulted from a strategy based on evidence which, when we look at it dispassionately, is totally compelling. One group of medical professionals examine a patient with dirty hands carrying pathogens; those in another group wash their hands before doing so. The mortality rate of the patients of the first group is much higher some days after examination than that of the second group. Therefore, see what difference it makes to patient mortality if the first group of doctors wash their hands. The intervention is simple and inexpensive, and any effect should be manifest in a short time.

We believe that the arguments we have made for the importance of development to the prevention of non-communicable disease globally are equally clear and compelling. Look at the map of deaths around the world from non-communicable diseases. It is dominated not by the West but by Asia. It will explode soon in other regions of the world. It is obvious that we won't be able to have much impact in Asia by merely applying the approaches we have used in the West— no more than strict adherence to the 'bad humours' theory of disease was able to prevent any deaths from infection in the wards where Semmelweis worked. The current approach is not working—people are dying. Something must have been overlooked.

We contend that what has been overlooked is development, in both senses of the word. For early life development and socio-economic development are not independent of each other: they interact and are interdependent. In statistics, when two processes interact we do not just add the two effects to assess the total effect— we multiply them together. Understanding the importance of this interaction, development multiplied by development, is a major missing piece in solving the puzzle of non-communicable disease.

Development in one dimension

Given that we are losing the war against obesity, diabetes, and cardio-vascular disease in the West, except by using intensive medical interventions, why should we imagine that our currently favoured strategies will work in the less developed world? The solution must lie in the broader development agenda and its increasing focus on education as a route to empowerment. We have at least one international agency which is increasingly taking the lead in this regard—the United Nations Development Programme. While this agency has traditionally focused on crisis situations such as famine, civil war, and earthquakes, increasingly its leadership is thinking about women's empowerment and education, child development, and gender equality. Focusing on the mother-to-be from a young age must be a priority even though in some cultures this will be very challenging. It will require insightful leadership at international, national, and local levels.

For reasons that we hope stand out from every page of this book, we hope that such programmes are reinforced and developed further. The United Nations Development Programme and its sister agencies including UN Women, now led by Michelle Bachelet, a former paediatrician and past president of the Republic of Chile, and the United Nations Children's Fund need to be engaged and supported in this battle. They may even play a more important role than the World Health Organization, because the problem is not simply medical. And the major non-governmental organizations and philanthropic donors need to play their role too. We remain very concerned that such agencies seem to have been largely excluded from defining the global strategy needed to win the war.

Development in the second dimension

Different people clearly have very different sensitivities to living in the obesogenic world which we have created. And it is now very clear that much of this difference is established so early in our lives that it is no longer right to say 'It is mainly your own fault' to people who are obese or who are developing chronic disease.

Genes explain some of this difference in sensitivity between individuals but not that much, and in any case we cannot do anything about our genes any more than we can choose our parents or rerun human evolution. But the ways in which we develop from a fertilized egg to a child depend on much more than our genes, and appear to influence a substantial component of our risk of developing non-communicable disease by priming us for how we will respond to the world as we grow up. Those developmental processes are moulded by the developmental environment, and we *can* do something about that.

Many factors operating before our birth can have enormous influences on our later health. Much of that effect is mediated by epigenetic processes and the science of unravelling this is advancing fast. It has revealed how the changes in gene switches induced by factors such as the mother's diet put some people more at risk later than others. We think this science will soon create new approaches to the problem—it will tell us much more about how to create a healthy start to life. It will shift the point of focus from adults to potential parents, to both mothers and fathers, and to their babies.

Developmental risk is not about extremes of birth size or extremes of maternal stress or food intakes. Rather our biology was set up tens of thousands of years ago for ensuring that we pass our genes on to the next generation, and the echoes of that biology restrict how we can now adjust to a new world, a world we never evolved to inhabit. Perhaps the most dramatic demonstration of those echoes is in the simple observation that first-born children are biologically different at birth from subsequent children, an observation with extraordinary implications for both Europe and China.

As we look at it in more detail, it becomes apparent that different developmental factors could play a significant role in different parts of the world. In India an important factor is constraint of fetal growth in stunted mothers. In much of the developing world the initiating factors may be poor maternal nutrition, often associated with heavy workloads in pregnancy, and maternal stress. In other places indoor pollution from cooking on smoky fires or charcoal, or pollution from traffic or industry, plays a major role. In still other places, such as urban China, it is the rapid increase in maternal obesity and gestational diabetes. Few of the 130 million births which occur each year will be unaffected by at least one of these factors.

Our development does not stop at birth. In our infancy and early childhood we learn eating habits from our parents, and some of these become hard-wired in our brains. Our food and taste preferences, our appetite controls, some metabolic settings, and possibly even the amount of exercise we are willing to undertake are all established in our brains in the first few months and years of our lives.

And the evidence is now accumulating fast that we can do things in early life that will make a difference—even if we have a way to go before we can be sure how effective these measures will be. Prolonged exclusive breastfeeding, appropriate maternal nutrition in pregnancy and lactation, and nutritional education for potential parents and young children are three simple measures that could be implemented in many parts of the world. They would have many other benefits as well, in reducing infant deaths and improving both maternal health and brain development in children.

Mixed emotions

In writing this book we have expressed on different pages emotions of frustration, excitement, and hope.

We are frustrated because it is manifestly obvious that we are failing to deal with one of the most important issues of our time—we are getting fatter in every country and are starting to see very high rates of non-communicable disease in some places. Even in some of the poorest parts of the developing world, where such disease is not yet common, nonetheless we see warning signs of its arrival. The burden of disease in the world is shifting from infectious to non-communicable disease, yet the resources spent on prevention of the former continue to far outweigh those spent on the latter. It is understandable and natural that we should focus our resources on acute problems, because that is only fair to those who are already sick, but in doing so we must be cognizant that life-course equity requires consideration of the prevention of what may happen in future years both at an individual and at a population level.

This issue of intergenerational equity is acute. We have seen it operate in the debate over climate change. Do we have to act now or can we afford to wait in the hope of a future technological solution? We see it in relation to non-communicable disease risk in the next generation. Should we wait and hope that they can solve this in their time?

And we are frustrated that the current strategy seems to be based on the operation of individual choice, which proved to be successful in the compaign against smoking. But does the little girl force-fed before marriage in rural Mauritania have any choice in her life? Does the 12-year-old child bride in rural India have any choice when she becomes pregnant and drops out of school? Does the little toddler in Detroit have any choice when his mother feeds him French fries? Does the little boy from Tonga whose mother had diabetes in pregnancy have any choice about developing obesity? Does the little boy in Beijing have any choice in being an only child? And yet every one of these scenarios, and many more, sets that little child up with a greater risk of becoming obese and suffering from a non-communicable disease. They are all matters beyond their control.

Obesity, diabetes, and cardiovascular disease are not the same thing. There are individual and population differences in the relationships between them and that complicates matters too, biologically and psychologically. But one thing is common to them all. They are all very slowly developing conditions, and so subtle changes in their development can nonetheless have substantial effects on health later. The early life changes can be so subtle that we may not know when they start, but that does not diminish their importance.

When does the problem go from being one of prevention to one of treatment? Pondering this, we start to get excited because our new scientific understanding reveals that what makes us what we are is a combination of our genes, how we developed from a single egg and sperm, and how we live in the modern world. This realization has been slow to be incorporated into the general scientific framework, impeded as it has been by the focus on the gene—but it is now undeniable. It is an exciting time for medical science.

Within this conceptual framework we are starting to uncover many things that will give us new tactics and strategies for the war against obesity and non-communicable disease, and so we are hopeful. We now know that we will have to give much greater attention to the mother and unborn child. We may well have to focus on the lifestyle of the father as well. And most importantly of all, we are starting to realize that behaviours such as the propensity to exercise, which we previously thought were based on individual choice, have a large constitutional component—based in part on inherited genes, in part on epigenetic changes to gene function in response to the developmental environment, and in part through early learning.

We now face a world where more people suffer from apparent over-nutrition rather than under-nutrition. But paradoxically both can lead to chronic disease. It may be better to think of it as unbalanced nutrition—nutrition mismatched to our evolved biology— affecting much of the world's population. These issues are growing in the developing world. When combined with climate change, issues of water, food, and energy security, changes in life expectancy and family size, as well as many other factors, the burden of non-communicable disease will truly add to the 'perfect storm' that we mentioned at the start of the book. We see the clouds gathering. Weathering this storm will require the combined effort of governments, agencies, foundations, and the private sector.

The world of the vain emperor, whose sycophantic advisers had assured him that his clothes were too fine to be seen, changed when the little boy exclaimed that the emperor had no clothes. Medicine changed when the significance of Semmelweis' work was eventually recognized. Across the world, we have not been well served by the current initiatives to prevent non-communicable disease. We are getting fat and we are dreadfully unhealthy. It is apparent that new strategies are needed if we are all to take the pathways to healthier lives. It is in the interests of all of us to listen to the little boy's cry.

Index